Praise for Bright Kids Who Couldn't Care Less

"Dr. Braaten distills research and decades of clinical experience into this hugely useful guide. The book throws a lifeline to parents struggling to understand a kid who seems to have given up. If you want to help children discover and enjoy their strengths, this book is a must read."

—Lisa Damour, PhD, author of *The Emotional Lives of Teenagers*

"Dr. Braaten's incredible commitment to eradicating the 'myth of lazy' shines through on every page. For our family, the book sensitively broke down issues that felt overwhelming. It provided clear, actionable steps that helped us reframe our children's challenges and focus on their strengths and talents instead."

—Ashley J., Coatesville, Pennsylvania

"If you're pulling out your hair in frustration as you watch your child not care—and not care about not caring—this book is for you. Before you lecture your child yet again, or worse, give up, Dr. Braaten has answers that work and are simple to use. With the skill of an experienced safecracker, she teaches you to unlock your child's world and open up dazzling possibilities. Wise, practical, savvy, and warm."

—Edward Hallowell, MD, coauthor of *ADHD 2.0*

"This is the book that any parent who has ever said, 'I don't understand how such a smart kid just doesn't care about doing well!' needs to read. It demystifies motivation and offers practical suggestions, guidance about appropriate expectations, and empathic advice. I wish I'd had this book when my own children were younger. Dr. Braaten empowers parents to help kids succeed, and, just as important, to let kids be partners in defining what success looks like."

—Amanda Morin, educational consultant
and author of *Adulting Made Easy*

"Dr. Braaten skillfully helps you understand where kids' motivation comes from and the complex factors that may cause difficulties. She also addresses a critical question: Are your expectations for your child a good fit for who they are and the future they want? Parents concerned about motivational issues will want to read this book!"

—Timothy E. Wilens, MD, coauthor of *Straight Talk about Psychiatric Medications for Kids*

Bright Kids Who Couldn't Care Less

Also Available

Bright Kids
Who Couldn't
Care Less

HOW TO REKINDLE
YOUR CHILD'S MOTIVATION

Ellen Braaten, PhD

Foreword by Sheryl Sandberg

THE GUILFORD PRESS

New York   London

Library of Congress Cataloging-in-Publication Data is available from the publisher.

ISBN 978-1-4625-4764-7 (paperback) — ISBN 978-1-4625-5165-1 (hardcover)

For Miguel Fernandez Mandek, who showed me
how to care more about everything at a time
when it would have been much easier for me to care less

Contents

Author's Note

In this book, I alternate among masculine, feminine, and plural pronouns when referring to a single individual. The intention behind this word choice is to represent as many readers as possible as our language continues to evolve. I sincerely hope that all will feel included.

All illustrations of families in this book are composites of individuals whose personal information, including demographic details, has been altered to protect their identities.

Foreword

As parents, we all have hopes and dreams for our children. We wish for them to be healthy, to discover what's truly meaningful to them, and to go after their goals. But our hopes and dreams aren't enough. For children to fulfill their potential, they need to find motivation from within. And as kids grow older and change, it can be hard for them to stay in touch with their internal drive.

It's heartbreaking to watch a child lose enthusiasm for the hobbies, interests, and friendships that once brought them joy. Dr. Ellen Braaten's *Bright Kids Who Couldn't Care Less* can help. It provides an in-depth look at why some children lose motivation and a practical guide for parents and teachers to light that fire again.

Too often, parents don't know where to turn if their child has lost enthusiasm for just about everything. They are left facing so many questions alone: How did a child whose eyes lit up when playing with the family pets or who spent hours practicing passes on the soccer field turn into one who has to be dragged out of bed? Why doesn't anything I say or do seem to get through to them? Is this lack of enthusiasm just a phase? Am I expecting too much of my child—or too little? What can I do to help my child grow up to be happy and successful?

As Ellen explains, motivation is complicated. It doesn't just spring up out of nowhere. Reigniting it requires close attention to the goals our children are passionate about and the barriers that are getting in the way of pursuing them. Fortunately, this book offers a straightforward explanation of how motivation works and a formula for helping get a child back on track—whether that means finding a new passion or rediscovering an old one.

Lifelong interests and abilities are often evident from a young age. But as kids grow, it's all too easy for parents to lose sight of those early signs. We sometimes develop such a sharp image of who our kids will be—or who we want them to be—that we forget to look closely at who they actually are. To help them reconnect to their passion, parents need to focus on what their children truly care about. We need to avoid "magical thinking"—the idea that our kids can do anything—and, instead, take an honest look at what they have the aptitude for and the ability to pursue. And we need to support them in setting reasonable goals and building the skills to achieve them.

Instilling in our children a love of discovery, learning, and accomplishment matters deeply. Not only does it lay the foundation for long-term growth and happiness, but it can also help children build their individual resilience. As our children grow, they'll undoubtedly face adversity. It's often motivation that will help them persevere during hardship and move forward with greater resolve. For example, during the COVID-19 pandemic, Ellen saw firsthand in her clinical practice that the children who knew what they were interested in and what they were good at were often less likely to get derailed by isolation and boredom. By tapping into intrinsic motivation, she was able to help countless children weather the challenges of the pandemic and emerge more grounded and determined.

This is a remarkable book by a remarkable woman. I've had the opportunity to see Ellen in action. A psychologist and researcher, she is a leader in the field of pediatric neuropsychological and psychological assessment. She has been a faculty member at Harvard Medical School for almost 25 years and is the founder and Executive Director of the Learning and Emotional Assessment Program at Massachusetts General Hospital—a nationally recognized center for evaluating learning differences.

Ellen cares deeply about empowering parents and helping them become stronger, more effective advocates for their children. For decades, she has counseled and provided therapy to families who have been lucky enough to see her. In *Bright Kids Who Couldn't Care Less*, Ellen's wisdom and expertise are now available to everyone. She shares dozens of strategies to get children back on track quickly, showing readers how to ensure that the children they care about know how to stay in touch with what drives them, whatever path they choose.

For parents who are struggling to motivate their children, this book will give you hope that your child can find their way to a happy, healthy future. It will teach you how to nurture your child's strengths, and it provides the tools you need to help them thrive again. For teachers fighting to keep their students on track, this book explains proven methods for setting clear, flexible goals and fostering a growth mindset. For anyone who cares about the next generation, this book is a gift.

SHERYL SANDBERG

Acknowledgments

This book would never have been published without the knowledge and insight from my editors and friends Kitty Moore and Chris Benton. They are extraordinary editors who constantly amaze me with their intuition and their ability to keep me focused (not an easy task). There was not a conversation with either of them that didn't begin and end with laughter, with quite a lot of insight sandwiched in between. Every book I've written for them has included as least one difficult life experience for one or more of us (this time it was a shared worldwide pandemic), along with quite a few joyful events. It's been an honor and my incredibly good fortune to have worked with these talented women through good times and those times best forgotten.

It was also my incredibly good fortune to have the assistance of Clara Beery over the two years it took to write this book. So much of Clara's insight and wisdom is on the pages of this book (along with her creativity in every illustration). She has my eternal thanks as she moves on to graduate school in psychology. I don't know how I will ever write another book without her help.

My colleagues at Massachusetts General Hospital are some of the best professionals in the world. I am grateful for their support. Dr. Sheila O'Keefe and Amanda Morin, thank you for your insightful comments and support throughout this process. Your expertise is priceless, but I value your friendship even more. Same goes for Darlene Maggio, who has done a million things to keep me on track and supported me in countless ways for over a decade.

To my family, especially my children, Hannah and Peter, thanks for being my first teachers about what it means to be a parent and for being the joys of my life. Having a daughter who is an editor is a big bonus for the writer. Not so much for the editor. Thank you, Hannah, for listening, for reading, and for your never-ending patience. Miguel, thank you for your support, your love, and cups of coffee that always seemed to appear just when I needed them. Petar, the newest member of the family, thank you for showing me that you would be a conscientious and loving husband to my daughter by repeatedly, somewhat anxiously, asking, "Is your mom done with the book yet?"

The idea for this book was conceived in 2019 during a sabbatical at Charles University in Prague, an opportunity that wouldn't have happened had it not been for the support of Drs. Michal Goetz and Radek Ptáček. You are the best of colleagues and even better friends. Your support came at just the right time in my life. *Díky moc* from the bottom of my heart.

I am beyond blessed to have the book's foreword written by Sheryl Sandberg, a woman I have admired since reading *Lean In* in 2013. There is no better champion of women's causes than Sheryl. You set the standard for what it means to be a working mother, a business leader, and a generous philanthropist. I am in awe of what you've accomplished. And I'm eternally grateful to you for lending your voice to my book and your support to my work.

Finally, the true inspiration for this book came from the parents and kids with whom I've had the privilege of working over the past 25 years. I am honored that you've entrusted me with your care, and I have a deep sense of gratitude for all I've learned from you.

Introduction

The idea for this book started sometime in 2019. At that time, I had been noticing a trend in my clinical practice—unmotivated kids who couldn't care less about things that kids generally care about. Many were teens and preteens, but some were as young as early elementary school students. The parents voiced a general concern that sounded something like this: "My child doesn't seem to care about anything." Or "I just can't seem to get my child motivated." Or "If it wasn't for video games, my kid would do nothing at all."

I thought that this trend might have had something to do with the focus of my practice. A few years before, I'd written a book with Brian Willoughby called *Bright Kids Who Can't Keep Up,* about kids who process and respond to information more slowly than others. I assumed that maybe what I was seeing was a skewed sample. Were kids who had slower processing speed making up a larger part of my practice? Perhaps these unmotivated kids were "kids who couldn't keep up," I thought to myself. When I actually looked at the makeup of my clinical work, I found my practice was more varied than just one kind of child. What I thought was a skewed sample was really the tip of the iceberg. As I started to analyze this trend toward what I would have called apathy, I found it didn't fit into a single category. It wasn't just kids who couldn't keep up. Or kids who were depressed. Or anxious. Or learning disabled. Or addicted to video games. It was a problem that appeared to cut across the spectrum of learning and emotional disorders and of development. Increasingly, kids were being referred to me who had no diagnosable disorder except for "I can't get him motivated" or "she just doesn't seem to care."

And then came 2020, the year of the great demotivator for all of us. Followed by 2021, which only increased our sense of loss, reinforced feelings of helplessness, and resulted in apathy, lethargy, and a *who cares?* attitude for many kids and adults. A book about a subset of kids who didn't care seemed to have a broader audience. Many kids were having difficulty finding a reason to be interested in much of anything.

I wrote this book to empower parents—those parents who are feeling hopeless, helpless, and worried about their child's future. When you've got a kid who doesn't care about much, helping them get back on track can feel like an impossible task. You are your child's first and best advocate, and it's easier to advocate or help when you know exactly what to do. However, this isn't a how-to book. Kids who have lost motivation and who don't care don't fit into a particular "box." "Not caring" isn't something like a reading disability that can be fixed with the right curriculum. It's not like experiencing anxiety, which can be treated by learning stress management skills. It's a complicated situation with many causes. But just because I can't provide you with one-size-fits-all specific techniques doesn't mean there is nothing you can do. Your influence starts with understanding your child and reflecting on what caused your child to lose interest in the first place. It also involves understanding yourself and your expectations. This knowledge provides the basis for setting goals and finding a path forward. There's a lot you can do, but it's going to take some reflection.

My approach is to explore the issue of *kids who couldn't care less* from many different vantage points. I start with helping you identity the problem—why is it that so many kids don't seem to care about anything? I identify the factors that are essential to motivation and help you think about how these factors are important in your child's development and life. You will gain a better understanding of your child's unique qualities (and maybe your own too) and learn how your expectations might be getting in the way of motivation (and how you can readjust them if needed). The book finishes with chapters on how to set goals and maintain motivation. At the end of every chapter are places where you can reflect (the section "What to Think About"), questions that can lead to discussions ("What to Talk About"), and suggestions that might help ("What to Do").

To get the most out of the book I suggest you start at the beginning and read it through. You might be tempted to first look at the section on setting goals because you're eager to find a list of things you can do now. That's okay, but don't make that your ending point. Though one of the biggest problems for kids who couldn't care less is a lack of goals, starting with goal setting can be counterproductive. Understanding the personal, family, and social factors that lead kids to give up on their goals and keep them (and you) from setting realistic ones should come first. The first two parts of this book orient you, the reader, to these important ideas.

Part I of this book, "Why Some Kids Couldn't Care Less," frames the problem and identifies terms we use to describe motivation. What is motivation, and how do we become motivated in the first place? Once you have an understanding of motivation, we will spend time talking about the factors that apply to your child's motivation (or lack of)—their abilities, the things that give them pleasure, and the things they tend to spend time doing. I call this the Parenting APP—which stands for *aptitude, pleasure,* and *practice.* We will explore each one of these issues in depth.

Part II puts ability, pleasure, and practice into the larger context of societal expectations as well as connecting these concepts to your child's individual personality style. It will guide you to explore how your child's unique qualities affect motivation. You'll assess whether and how your expectations might get in the way of motivation and how to use expectations to help your child care more. You'll also find ideas about how to adjust your natural parenting style to fit the child you have. Along the way, I'll discuss the things, like college preparation and school–child fit, that get in the way of establishing well-chosen goals.

Part III is all about looking toward the future, with an emphasis on setting goals that are appropriate for your child. You'll learn why happiness (a goal of most parents) isn't really a goal in itself but the outcome of reaching good goals. You'll also find out that goals aren't the endpoint. They're the beginning of the journey. They're a road map for where you're going, and that journey will likely change in the process. Part III covers these issues too.

After reading the book, you might find you have many more questions that weren't answered here. In fact, you should have more questions. Continuing to learn more about your child's unique qualities and challenges will help you set good goals and revise them into better goals when necessary. Exploring topics like sleep schedules, social media, and learning differences (things only mentioned briefly in the book) might be helpful. Part IV offers more help should you need it. In Chapter 11, I provide some important information about when to worry if there's more than just a "don't care attitude" that's affecting your child. And in Chapter 12, you'll find some of my favorite books and websites on topics related to motivation but for which there was no space here.

Don't ever worry alone. Talk about your concerns with your child's pediatrician, teachers, and other adults who care for your child. Above all, don't feel hopeless—at least not for very long. While there's no easy "cure" for the child who "couldn't care less," this book, at the very least, should help you understand your child and the factors that are causing them to feel and behave this way. I believe understanding is the foundation of hopefulness. It is my wish that you find reasons to be hopeful in the pages of this book.

PART I

Why Some Kids Couldn't Care Less

ONE

"Why Doesn't My Bright Kid Seem to Care about Anything?"

"Excuse my language" was the first thing Bradley's father, Don, said to me when I asked him and his wife, Sandra, how I could be helpful.

"We came here to see you because Bradley doesn't give a crap about anything. He's not making it in school. But forget about school. Forget about passing ninth grade. The kid's flunking life. I don't care if he doesn't get into Harvard; I just don't want him living in my basement playing video games when he's 30."

"It's probably my fault," Sandra added. "I spoil him, but he does better if I help him. Especially in school. He could never keep up if I wasn't around."

"Help him?" Don replied. "You do the homework for him, and that's after paying for all the tutoring he's getting—Spanish, math, an executive function coach—whatever that is—we're doing everything for him. Probably way too much. You're right. He's spoiled. It's never his fault—and you let him get away with it. Listen, we've been to a lot of professionals, Doctor, and we've tried everything. Tutoring. Therapy. I tried to get him interested in hockey. Soccer. Nothing works. What's wrong with my kid? Can you do anything to help?"

Bradley's parents represent hundreds of families I've worked with over the last 25 years—parents of kids who, to paraphrase Bradley's dad, *couldn't care less about anything.* Parents will wonder "Is he lazy? Spoiled? Afraid to fail? Unmotivated? Gifted?" For some parents, it can start with a nagging feeling soon after their child starts school. They might tell me that their child never seemed that enthusiastic about anything to do with learning. Other parents, especially those of teens, notice a more recent lack of consistent passion for almost everything—friendships, home life, extracurricular activities. As kids grow, these minor problems develop into more serious issues. A child who fails to enjoy learning new things becomes one who stops doing his homework. Then he progresses to one whose grades are failing. Finally, he becomes the child who can't get off the couch.

Kids like Bradley sound remarkably similar, but the reasons for their behaviors rarely are. These behaviors, which one father aptly described to me as *malaizy*—a combination of malaise and lazy—all involve a lack of motivation, a diminished interest in things kids their age are typically interested in, and problems completing almost anything. This sounds on the surface like depression. And sometimes these kids are depressed. Often they are not. And even when depression is a factor, it's typically more complicated than just treating the biological symptoms of depression.

Kids who couldn't care less might look like they're malaizy—a combination of malaise and lazy.

Younger kids usually show fewer symptoms. They can keep up well enough in school or have a robust group of friends, but they might sometimes seem like much of life is boring to them. They might have difficulties completing homework or complain about participating in sports. Older kids typically show more concerning symptoms. Their boredom has become real malaise. They skip school. Fail to do any work independently. Check out of family activities and stop hanging out with friends, unless it's through social media or gaming. Alcohol and drug use can be a way to cope. Their *malaiziness*—at least at the beginning—can seem like a problem with motivation. As they get older, it can seem like severe depression or anxiety. In the middle of those extremes are many possible causes. Regardless of the cause or the age of the child, parents almost always bring up two words—*motivation* and *laziness*. Both of these concepts are important in understanding kids who couldn't care less. Let's start with motivation.

What Is Motivation?

Motivation is the *why* or the *reason* we do things. For example, we are motivated to get off the couch and get a glass of water because we are thirsty. But, even though we are *really* thirsty, we might not be motivated to get it ourselves if we can say to someone, "Hey, I'm thirsty. Can you get me something to drink?" and they do it. We tend to think that motivation is something that is built into us—like a single character trait—but it's really much more complicated and multifaceted. It's also affected, both positively and negatively, by the supports around us. If there is no one around us to get us the glass of water, we have no choice but to get it ourselves, so we are motivated to move rather than be motivated to ask someone to do it for us. And, if there's no water at all to be had in the house, things become complicated. We might be motivated to call a plumber, or we might feel completely discouraged because it all seems too overwhelming and we lose motivation entirely.

This simple example illustrates that we're not just talking about one thing when we are talking about motivation. It's not just desire or willpower. In fact, science has shown us that a number of factors underlie motivation: our biology, our emotions, our thoughts, and the social world in which we live. It's the *why* we do the things that we do, and that's something that is different for everyone—and it can change over time and because of circumstances.

No single theory explains everything about the complexity of motivation.

Psychologists have spent years studying and developing theories about motivation. No single theory explains everything about the complexity of the topic. It's important to keep this in mind when you've got a child who seems unmotivated. Thinking about it from many different perspectives will be important. Here are some of the most widely accepted theories of motivation. Think about each one of these and how it may or may not relate to your child.

THEORIES OF MOTIVATION

The *instinct theory of motivation* is based on the fact that all of us are born with innate biological tendencies—or *instincts*—that help us survive. Babies are born with reflexes, like the rooting reflex, which causes them to begin sucking and turn toward a food source when their cheeks or lips are touched. Birds fly south for the winter. We seek shelter when it's raining and warmth when we're cold. Maternal instinct is considered a built-in readiness that most women have toward mothering. This theory states that all humans have the same motivations because we all generally have the same biology. Thus, the root of all motivations is the motivation to survive.

You can probably see there are problems with this theory. Not every mother is maternal. We aren't birds. Our preprogrammed motivations are subject to individual experiences and emotions like jealousy and desire. But biology factors into some things. In terms of your child's behavior: *think about the role of biology and how it might relate to your child's difficulties.* It won't explain all the reasons he couldn't care less, but it might give you insight into some basic ones.

Incentive theory explains that people are motivated to do things because of external rewards. For example, adults are motivated to go to work every day because they want to receive a paycheck. For kids, incentives would include good grades for studying, getting praised for behaving well, or getting paid for doing chores. In Chapter 5, I'll talk a lot about how incentives can sometimes undermine kids' motivation. For now, *think about the incentives that work for your child.* Not all incentives are created equally, and the rewards that you find motivating might not be the same ones your child finds appealing.

Sometimes our motivation is affected by our need to reduce internal tension. That's the idea behind the *drive theory of motivation.* For example, we are motivated to cook something to reduce the internal state of hunger. Alternatively, a child might be motivated to complete—or even *not complete*—a homework assignment because the teacher will be angry if the homework isn't completed (in the first case) or because the child is afraid he can't complete the assignment correctly. The tension and embarrassment of turning in a poor assignment and looking "stupid" is worse than the tension of having an irate teacher (second case). *Are there instances where your child seems driven to act in a certain way to reduce tension?* If your child has difficulty completing homework independently, and little possibility of getting rewarded for what he is able to do without your support, he might be motivated *not* to do tasks that you think he should be doing. He might be motivated to let you do them for him.

The *arousal theory of motivation* is all about maintaining our psychological status quo. Arousal, in this case, is about our desire not to be too out of control or too "on edge," but also not to be too bored or lethargic. We tend to feel best in the middle. This theory of motivation suggests that people take certain actions to either decrease or increase levels of arousal, so that we are in that middle zone. We watch an exciting TV show when we are bored or take a bath or meditate when our arousal levels are high. Kids often "check out" by playing video games or overdoing it on social media when they are feeling overwhelmed. They might gravitate toward dangerous behavior when they are bored or lack a purpose. *What kind of things does your child tend to do when bored or overwhelmed?* These can be potential motivators or destroyers of motivation.

Other theories, like the one speculated by Abraham Maslow in the 1940s, says that we need to fulfill certain basic needs before other, more psychological needs; see the diagram on page 12. At the bottom of the hierarchy are basic needs like food and water. On top of that are needs like being safe and secure. Belongingness and "love needs" like friendship and intimate relationships are important as we move up the pyramid, followed by esteem needs (like prestige and a feeling of accomplishment) and, finally, self-actualization (achieving one's full potential). According to this theory, for motivation to arise at the next stage, the needs at each lower stage must be satisfied. This is an important concept to consider, because we often expect kids to be at the stage of self-actualization—and to be motivated by that factor—when they haven't yet had their needs for belongingness or a sense of accomplishment satisfied. Maslow's theory mostly referred to development over a lifetime, but the needs on this pyramid occur on a daily basis too, like when a child is too hungry or tired to concentrate on his

Maslow's Hierarchy of Needs

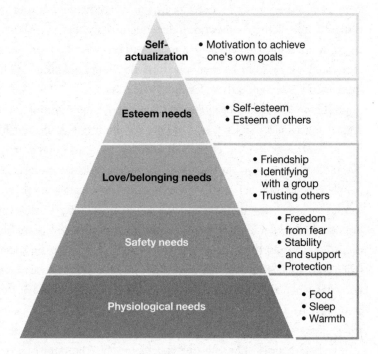

HOW MASLOW'S PYRAMID LOOKS IN CHILDREN

- Physiological needs: Kids always need to be well rested, well fed, and warm before anything else. So even highly motivated children will have trouble being motivated to tackle a difficult task if they slept poorly the night before.

- Safety needs: Freedom from fear and instability comes next. For example, a child who focuses primarily on avoiding punishment may struggle to develop intrinsic motivation, or any motivation at all.

- Love/belonging needs: Just like adults, kids who lack strong friendships or a sense of belonging may be less motivated because they have neither a base of support nor a source of identity.

- Esteem needs: Children need to know what their strengths are and see them celebrated by others to form a strong self-concept; without that they will struggle to develop motivation.

homework. *Where is your child on this hierarchy? Are there needs that aren't met that might be impeding motivation? Are there needs, like enough sleep or supportive friendships, that are tough to satisfy on a daily basis?* These categories aren't firm. In fact, self-actualization is a lifelong process, but sometimes kids get stuck in one category of needs. For example, when a child is having difficulty forming friendships, it is hard to move up the pyramid and be motivated by prestige and a feeling of accomplishment.

Speaking of not getting needs met, you're probably wondering if stress is behind your child's lack of motivation; see the sidebar on pages 14–15.

Finally, *expectancy theory* is all about the future—we are motivated to do certain things because we expect the effort will lead to better performance, which will in turn lead to better rewards. This is very dependent on how we view the future and formulate different predictions. *Do I have control over the future?* If yes, we are more motivated. *Do I value what is likely to happen in the future?* If yes, we're more motivated. If we don't value it, we're not very motivated. *Do I have the skills to produce the outcome that is expected of me?* If not, we can't expect success and thus aren't very motivated to even try.

There is not a better example for expectancy theory than the college admission process. This is such an important topic that I will explore it in depth in Chapter 8. The expectation for college starts long before high school. It's not always a realistic motivator. It's often not the best motivator. For kids who struggle in school, it can be a demotivator—something off in the future that is scary. If everyone expects you to go to college and you know you don't have the skills for it, or if you want a career that doesn't require a college degree, you are not motivated by this expectation. In fact, if you're a high school student, you might be motivated to act out. You might skip class or not turn in assignments.

Yael was one of these kids. From the time she was 12, she had wanted to be a hairstylist and makeup artist.

"Sure, you can do that," her parents would tell her. "Once you finish college. Everyone needs a college degree first."

Yael didn't see the point, and she was right. She didn't love school. She loved fashion. She didn't read novels, but she spent a lot of time reading

Could It Just Be Too Much Stress?

Stress is one reason some kids give up and lose their way. Some of these kids were high achievers from an early age—the spelling bee champion in second grade, the captain of the science team in middle school. By 10th grade they're tired and worn out. Some start drinking or smoking weed. Others begin underperforming. Address this issue head on, by asking what happened and fixing the things you can change. The things to think about, talk about, and do at the end of each chapter can help guide your discussions. Therapy can also be helpful, as can decreasing the level of stress.

In fact, decreasing stress will help *all* kids stay on track, even if they were never high achievers. One of the greatest sources of stress occurs when we feel we have no control over our lives. It can be something as simple as realizing you don't have enough time to complete the homework before it's due or as complex as having an untreated learning disability, which can make most aspects of school feel out of your control. Racial inequality, poverty, medical problems, and learning differences can be sources of chronic stress, while unexpected disasters can interfere in a child's development and produce problems in adjustment.

The COVID-19 pandemic was occurring while I was writing this book, and it will take quite some time for us to understand the effects of this stressful event on children and families. Studies of children who have faced other disasters, from 9/11 to tsunamis, have shown that the likelihood that a child will face problems following a disaster depends on factors such as the nature of the disaster, its severity, and the support available to the child. What the parent experiences after a disaster plays an important role in how the child will respond. In terms of COVID-19, everyone suffered some, many suffered a lot. It's taking time for things to get back to normal, even if your family was lucky enough to never experience significant illness or death. If your experience was much more severe, it might take you more time to feel like you are back on track—and the tracks might lead somewhere you didn't expect. Give yourself—and your child—time to heal. What are some other things you can do?

- In a crisis, kids want to know the answer to three things: Am I safe? Are the people I love safe? How will my life change because of this situation? You might not know the answers to all of these questions, but you can say things like "We are doing all we can to stay safe" and "Here's what we're planning to do to get through."

- In addition to keeping those questions in mind, reassure children (many times if necessary) about their safety and security.

- Allow kids to talk about their stress and the events they experienced, and be patient and nonjudgmental when listening to them.

- In general, don't expose kids to more stress than they already have. If there's a frightening news event, limit discussions to what's appropriate for them to know at their age. Answer their questions, but don't have the news blaring all day when it's a string of frightening events.

- Help kids make sense of what happened. If it was a traumatic event, make sure they don't think they caused it. For example, a child might think she caused her mom's cancer because she said "I hate you, Mommy!" when she was in kindergarten. Another child might think Grandma died from COVID-19 because he didn't wash his hands enough. Other kids might believe things happened that didn't. Slowly help them develop a realistic understanding of the important, stressful events in their lives.

- If your child's stress is less about a traumatic experience and more about the chronic stress of homework, social relationships, and overworked parents, the same advice applies. Even very smart high school students have unrealistic ideas. They might think that getting a B+ on a test will make them ineligible to be accepted at Yale, or that if they don't win the tennis championship, "no college will want me." Talk to them realistically about how college acceptance isn't about one test or accomplishment. It might also be helpful to let them know that a lot about college admissions is outside their control. Yet it's been my experience that kids who are motivated to go to college—and who understand that a lot of the process lies outside their control—are generally very happy with where they ultimately attend school. This is especially true if they've been able to manage the stressors of high school by learning to enjoy the process and to not focus too much on the goal, which happens to be another way to manage stress.

Vogue and *Glamour* and researching fashion trends. She was a passionate student and a hard worker at the hair salon where she was employed on Saturday mornings. As the deadline for college applications approached, she started skipping classes and avoided doing homework. She had clearly told her parents what she wanted with her words and actions. But when they didn't listen—when their goals didn't match hers—she went from a child who was motivated to be successful at her chosen profession to one who was motivated to show her parents in a most difficult way that college wasn't her choice, by becoming an unmotivated high school senior who was in jeopardy of not graduating.

"How can I motivate him? How can I get him to care?" parents will ask me, as if there is a series of steps that can fix the problem. As you can see, it's complicated. The downside is that there isn't a simple solution, but the upside is that there are unlimited places to intervene and make a difference. But before you can intervene, you have to know exactly what the problem is.

Components of Motivation

All of the theories of motivation assume that there are at least three major components to motivation:

● *Initiation.* The decision to begin an activity or behavior. It's the ability to get started on a task. Kids with poor initiation might look like they just don't want to do the work or that they are disinterested. Typically, though, they want to succeed but don't know how to get started. If your child struggles with initiation, you might find that your child has trouble getting started on homework or chores, along with a need for lots of reminding (you might describe it as nagging) to get started.

● *Persistence.* The effort we put toward continuing to try to reach a goal, even if obstacles stand in our way. It's our ability to continue to try, even when we experience frustrations or failures. Kids who are motivated stick with a task long enough to finish it. Persistence requires the ability to self-monitor, or be aware of where we are in the process. It requires good attention skills and the ability to not get distracted.

• *Intensity.* The concentration and stamina that go into pursuing a goal. It also includes the ability for students to assess their own performance while working on a task so that they can judge how much more work (intensity) the task requires.

All of these elements of motivation require executive function skills. *Executive function skills* are the skills that help us plan and achieve our goals. These skills include the ability to be flexible when thinking, self-monitor, pay attention, inhibit impulses, remember what you're supposed to do and when you're supposed to do it, manage your time, and stay organized. Kids who have difficulties with executive function skills have trouble with motivation, because they lack the skills to be motivated.

It's important to consider each one of these areas when you're evaluating your child's behavior. *Is she having difficulty getting started (initiation)? Sticking with it (persistence)? Or does she show a lack of attention and passion (intensity)?* Obviously, it can be all three, but sometimes one is a more chronic problem than the others and, when it is, it can be a useful place to start a conversation: "I saw that you were excited to start the project your teacher assigned—making a comic book about an event in history—and I know the topic you picked, last year's Super Bowl, is something you're passionate about. So what's getting in the way of getting it done? What do you need and what can I do to help?"

> Which component seems to be the biggest problem for your child—getting started, sticking with tasks, or concentrating and reviewing how the work is going?

In addition, it's good to get a sense of your child's executive function skills and how they might be getting in the way of motivation. There are a lot of good books on this topic (see the resources in Chapter 12 for more ideas). If you're really concerned about this, an assessment can be helpful in determining your child's executive function skills. See Chapter 11.

What Does an Unmotivated Child Look Like? Because Where I Come from, We Call It "Lazy"

Yael's lack of motivation was an easy one to spot and a relatively easy one to fix once her parents learned to accept and value Yael's abilities and goals for her life. It's usually not that simple. Remember Bradley? The roots of his lack of motivation and tendency not to care started earlier in childhood. In preschool, he had difficulty staying focused and his teacher described him as a bit "lethargic." In fact, his teacher frequently wondered if he was getting enough sleep at night. By second grade, he was diagnosed with attention-deficit/hyperactivity disorder (ADHD)—inattentive type and slow processing speed. School was difficult for him because he had trouble paying attention and it took him longer to do things than it did the average child. Although he received support services at school, they were never enough. At different times in his life, he displayed all of the symptoms in the chart on the facing page. By the time he was in his first year of high school, years of being told he was lazy had taken a toll on his self-esteem. He was discouraged and demoralized. He was experiencing something called *learned helplessness*—the idea that after having many similar adverse experiences we learn either to avoid those experiences or to become dependent on others, even when we have the ability to do something on our own. Bradley often did both. He avoided anything that smacked of hard work and relied on his mother's support to do things like writing assignments and studying for tests, even when he possessed the skill to do them himself. He lacked *persistence* and *resilience*. See the table on page 19 for signs of lack of motivation at different ages.

Although Bradley's parents were eager for me to give them answers, I did the opposite. I started by asking them questions to help them—and me—know exactly what we were talking about. When you've got a child like Bradley, it feels like nothing is working and everything has gone wrong. It can feel that way because the problem is poorly defined. When the problem is "he's lazy," or "he doesn't seem to care about anything," it can feel overwhelming because we don't have treatments for laziness or "not caring."

SIGNS OF AN UNMOTIVATED CHILD

Age 5–8	9–13	14–18	Young adults
• Has trouble doing things on her own • Says things like "I'm dumb" or "Reading is stupid" • When something doesn't go their way, they struggle to bounce back • Frequent temper tantrums • Can't organize even simple tasks or consistently follow directions • Requires parent involvement beyond the age where it's appropriate • Refuses to do schoolwork	• Complains a lot about being bored and can't entertain himself • Starts to say "I'm bad at" or "I can't do" a specific academic subject or activity • Says "It doesn't even matter if I try" • Has trouble deciding what she wants to do because nothing seems that interesting • Is overly sensitive to criticism • Complains that teachers are "unfair" or "stupid" • Doesn't complete homework assignments	• Struggles to come up with longer-term goals and follow through on steps • Struggles to identify any activities that interest them • Has no meaningful education or career goals, is uninterested in the college process, or says "I want to go to college," but doesn't do the work that it would take to reach that goal • Spends more time hanging out with other seemingly unmotivated students • Withdraws from competitive situations, even ones, such as sports, that used to be fun • May use drugs or alcohol as a way to "cope" • Obsessive video game playing • Frequently late for class	• Doesn't try to solve workplace or university problems independently, asks for help immediately • Hides bad grades or other perceived "failures" from others • Frequent lying • Difficulty forming and keeping relationships • Frequently late for work or class

At any age

- Procrastinates on homework and projects until the last minute
- Attributes any successes to luck, rather than their own skills and abilities
- Abandons an activity after a failure
- Avoids difficult academic tasks
- Doesn't try new activities
- Doesn't ask for help when things are too hard
- Asks for help before trying something independently
- Avoids nonpreferred tasks that could help them accomplish goals
- Gives up on new ideas quickly
- Has feelings of anxiety or depression
- Has an attitude of "I don't care" or "It doesn't matter"
- Follows the crowd, to the exclusion of developing their own interests
- Doesn't do self-care that is appropriate for his age, from hanging up coat to remembering to take lunch to school

The symptoms of **ADHD** are *inattention, impulsivity,* and *hyperactivity.* There are three types or presentations of ADHD—kids can be *primarily impulsive/hyperactive, primarily inattentive,* or a *combination of hyperactive/impulsive and inattentive.* The most common presentation is *ADHD-combined.*

Processing speed is the pace at which we take in information, make sense of it, and generate a response. In other words, how long it takes us to get something done, whether it be answering a question like "What do you want for breakfast?" or writing an essay.

Learned helplessness is the idea that, after many exposures to adversity, some people may stop trying to avoid those negative experiences and simply "give up." A good example of this in children is when they learn to be dependent on others, despite the ability to complete the tasks themselves.

Resilience is our ability to recover, and even grow, from difficult or stressful events. There's a lot more about resilience in Chapter 10, where I talk about developing a growth mindset, as well as further reading about the topic listed in Chapter 12.

But we do have treatments and solutions for the underlying reasons for those behaviors. We just have to start defining what those behaviors and triggers are. Other chapters in this book will look at these factors, such as skill deficits, family factors, and parental expectations, in depth, but let's start by thinking about the following questions. You might even want to get out a notebook and write your answers down.

My child couldn't care less. What exactly is it that he "doesn't care about"?

Define the things your child doesn't care about. You might think it's "everything." Maybe it is, but you won't know until you write them all down: School. Friends. His little sister. Family mealtimes.

If you found yourself writing broad categories, like "school," be more specific: Reading chapter books. Math. Ms. Burrow's Spanish class. Whatever it is, it's important to be clear.

How do I know she doesn't care?

What behaviors is your child exhibiting that make you know she doesn't care? Tantrums. Never leaves her room. Doesn't do her math homework. Never wants a friend over for a playdate. Write all of them down and "star" the ones that are most traumatic for you and the most problematic for her. They might not be the same.

Are my expectations reasonable for my child?

Take a look at the table on page 22. While these are only general guidelines for different ages—and only provide a few examples for each age group—they are good starting points to consider. Where do your expectations fall on these important markers of development? Are your expectations too high? Are your expectations so low that you no longer have any?

Are there changes at home or at school that might be causing or contributing to these behaviors?

Things like a new school, a parent's illness, a new sibling, or almost any change can affect motivation. Rarely is a change ever the entire problem, but it's important to label it and consider if it is part of the problem.

Are there social factors that might be a consideration?

Bullying, the loss of a best friend, a particularly "mean class," and the lack of a supportive peer group are the "silent killers" of motivation. They're often "silent" because parents can sometimes be the last to know when kids are struggling socially. You might be aware of some of these, or you might want to do some checking in with your child or his teacher. Kids often aren't forthcoming when it comes to peer relationships, so you might need to ask some open-ended questions like the ones on page 23. Also see the sidebar on pages 23–24.

Age	Friendships	Academic behaviors	Home/self-care	Fully independent behaviors
5–7	Takes turns Goes on playdates without parent	Remembers important dates (field trips, dress-up days)	Does simple chores (for example, putting out cups on the table, putting away toys, feeding the dog) Takes off shoes	Able to put self to sleep
8–10	Leads activities when friends come over Goes on sleepovers without parent	Displays beginner time management skills (for example, knows they need to finish something by a certain time and starts early)	Packs a bag for school Chooses weather-appropriate clothing Does multistep unsupervised chores (for example, taking out the recycling, setting the table)	Walks to school or friend's home by self Puts food in the microwave/gets own snack
11–13	Schedules own time with friends Solves simple interpersonal issues	Completes multistep academic projects Keeps track of quizzes and tests	Packs own lunch Picks up room	Able to stay home alone Able to do "odd jobs" independently ● Mow the lawn ● Watch a younger sibling
14–18	Makes multistage plans with friends	Studies ahead of time for quizzes and tests	Able (although it may be a struggle) to keep room clean	Able to hold a job for pay
Young adults	Solves complex interpersonal issues	Manages the demands of multiple responsibilities	Cleans own dorm/apartment; does own laundry	Able to live independently with only necessary support from parents, such as paying for college

How to Get Your Kids to Open Up about Their Friendships

It can be very difficult to know what your child is doing with her friends. This is normal. Kids need to have a social life outside the family system. But not knowing anything isn't great because parents can help when things get tough. Sometimes it's easiest to ask about *other* kids. Kids would rather talk about how their friends are doing than about themselves. Their answers can give you some ideas about what is going on with them. Here are some things to keep in mind:

- Kids often don't like responding to direct questions from their parents, especially when it comes to sensitive subjects. Instead of asking a direct question such as "Are you being bullied?" ask it indirectly: "I've been hearing so much about bullying. Is it a big deal at your school?" or "What would you do if you were bullied?" Framing it this way can be an entrance into a more personal conversation.

- Be prepared to listen. This can be tough, especially when you think you could solve the problem for your child. Bite your tongue and listen.

- When you're not listening, ask open-ended questions: "How did you feel when she said that?" "What do you think Suzy should have done when that happened to her?" "How do you think this is going to turn out?" "What would you like to see happen?"

- Empathize. Being a kid is tough. Let them know you understand: "I can't believe Tom would say that to you. That must have felt horrible." "I can't believe you rode the bus the rest of the week after that happened. You're really brave." "I'm so sad that happened."

- Ask how you can help rather than jumping in to fix something. "What do you need from me?" and "Do you need help coming up with a solution?" are good ways of offering support.

- Talk in hypotheticals when you're watching a TV show or movie about friendships, bullying, stress, or subjects relevant to kids. This can provide a platform for discussing tough topics. It can also give you the excuse to share your own experiences in an empathic way. "That movie was so good, but the main character was under so much stress in school. Things were easier when I was her age. Is that really what it's like for you and your friends?" Or "I remember when I was in sixth grade. Just like in the movie, my friend Connie found a new best friend and they were so mean to me. I cried every night before I went to sleep for weeks."

Is there a skills deficit?

If your child has been evaluated for a learning or attention issue, you may already know that there is a problem with a specific area of academics that makes some aspects of school more difficult. If a child is struggling to read, it's hard to stay motivated in a classroom where all of the other students are reading at or above grade level. If you're not sure whether a skills deficit is an issue, it might be a good idea to get an evaluation to determine whether there is a specific problem that underlies the tendency not to care. There's more information about this in Chapter 11.

Is there an identifiable emotional issue?

An emotional disorder, such as anxiety or depression, might be a contributing factor. I discuss these issues in more detail elsewhere. For now, it's important to keep in mind that for some kids reversing not caring isn't just about trying harder or finding the right motivator. Anxiety and depression, by definition, will cause behaviors that will look like inertia or poor motivation. It's important to consider whether these might be an issue for your child, because the treatment will need to address them. The good news is that treatments such as therapy and medication are quite effective at addressing psychological disorders such as anxiety and depression.

What about Bradley?

Remember Bradley from the beginning of this chapter? I wrapped up my initial appointment with his parents with their feeling relieved that I understood their concerns but frustrated that I didn't have a succinct answer as to how to fix them. After reading this chapter, you might be feeling the same way. It is incredibly frustrating that there isn't a program or a medication that has been proven to solve the problematic behaviors that Bradley exhibits. But I think that one of the reasons kids like Bradley are becoming more common is that we live in a culture where we assume there is a solution for everything. When one solution doesn't work perfectly, some families feel like failures and mistrust schools or professionals. Other families shop around for a diagnosis. Some fault teachers. I can't blame them. People like me— mental health professionals, educators, medical doctors—have given them the idea that a list of goals and objectives or the right medication will fix the issue. Don't get me wrong. We have terrific medications and psychological treatments for kids. But they have limits. And kids change. What worked in second grade doesn't necessarily work in sixth.

When Bradley was diagnosed with ADHD in second grade, his parents and teachers thought medication would be the solution to his problems. Medication and an individualized education program (IEP) definitely helped, but as Bradley matured, so did his vulnerabilities. And the effects of his vulnerabilities were subtle and difficult to see. The medication stopped working well after he had a growth spurt in middle school, and Bradley complained about taking pills. Instead of trying a new prescription and discussing why he didn't like taking pills, his family gave up on medication. The IEP that gave Bradley the necessary support in elementary school was changed to a Section 504 plan in seventh grade because he was "doing so well and needs to take more initiative for his own learning." It took almost two years of school before it was obvious that he wasn't ready, at age 12, to take more initiative. He still needed support. The stress of having a child who wasn't doing well in school took a toll on Bradley's parents' marriage, and their constant arguing made him stressed and anxious. It was a never-ending cycle that none of them could stop.

As I ended the initial session with Bradley's parents, I pointed out that there were lots of reasons they were in my office. It wasn't just (to use Bradley's father's words) "My kid doesn't give a crap" but (also in Bradley's father's words) more like this:

"So, what you're saying, Doc, is that he's not just lazy. I still think he's a bit lazy, but I hear what you're saying. There are a bunch of things that he needs, and it might take us some time to figure them out. Some are because of him (that's where I think the laziness comes in), and some are because of us (that's where I think my wife comes in), and some have to do with the school situation. We aren't going to fix this until we take a look at everything. Maybe even medication again. Okay. So, what's the next step?"

There were a lot of ways I could have answered this question. I could have started by pointing out that Don, Bradley's dad, was quick to put the blame on others, but in the moment that wouldn't have been helpful. I could have also sent them home with a list of things they needed to do right away—get a school or neuropsychological evaluation, get a consultation with a psychiatrist, convene a meeting with the school to discuss getting Bradley more support—and while I mentioned that they should consider doing all of these things at some point, I told them that first I'd like to meet with Bradley. The one thing that was missing from this initial appointment was Bradley's perspective. What were the personality or psychological factors that caused him to look like he couldn't care less? Those factors—the personal obstacles and characteristics like aptitude, pleasure, and temperament—are explored in the next few chapters.

THINK, TALK, DO

As I mentioned in the Introduction, at the end of each chapter, I'll provide you with action items to *think about,* to *talk about,* and to *do.* These suggestions are not an exhaustive list, but are a way to put into practice some of the topics discussed in the chapter and to make them more personal and meaningful for you.

What to Think About

- Why did you decide to read this book? What do you hope to learn about your child? What might you be afraid of knowing or thinking about?

- What are your fears about whether biological or genetic issues might be causing your child to act this way? Is there a history of anxiety, depression, or other mental health issues in your family that makes this more painful for you? How could you use this information to better understand your child?

- Are there recent changes in your child's life that might be contributing to a lack of motivation? If so, identify them, and if there are things that you can do to make these changes easier, list them as an action item in the "Do" section (see below).

- Where is your child on Maslow's hierarchy? Where is your family? Are there needs that are going unmet for your child or other members of your family that can be addressed? If so, make them action items in the "Do" section.

- Is your child having difficulty getting started (initiation)? Sticking with it (persistence)? Or does she show a lack of attention and passion (intensity)? If it seems to be more of one of these, that's a good place to start intervening. If it's all three, that's okay. It just means you need to take into account all of these things when figuring out future steps.

What to Talk About

- Ask your child to think about the motivators that work for her. Start the conversation clearly—"I want to know how best I can support you. Tell me some activities or rewards that would encourage you to get your homework done on time [or fill in the blank with whatever your child isn't doing]."

- Ask "What are the things that cause you to feel discouraged?"

- Open up a conversation about their friends or other kids you've observed (for better or worse). Phrases like "I noticed you've been hanging out with Desmond a lot lately. What's he like?" can be a good place to start. Try your best not to be judgmental or to stereotype kids. Approach it from a standpoint of wanting to know more. Rather than say "I'm not a fan of Desmond's tattoo. Sixteen is too young to get a tattoo," say "I noticed Desmond has a tattoo. What do you think of tattoos?"

What to Do

- Make a list of the exact things your child "doesn't care about."

- Make a list of the behaviors that show you that your child doesn't seem to care.

- Look at the two lists and star the one that bothers you the most. Check the one that seems to be most problematic for your child. Are they the same? If not, you'll want to start by addressing both of these.

- If you're concerned that your child is lacking the skills to be successful, talk to your child's teacher to get more information. Consider getting an evaluation of your child to determine whether a learning disability, attentional, or emotional issue could be leading to a lack of motivation. Keep in mind that *knowing* this, while scary, is the first step in finding a way to treat these issues.

TWO

The Parenting APP for Motivating Kids

APTITUDE, PLEASURE, AND PRACTICE

The motivation to learn about the world around us begins in infancy. Most parents have no difficulty encouraging a child's natural motivation when their children are babies or toddlers. We cheer on the child who is beginning to walk and persuade kids to climb to the top of the slide and come down. Encouraging motivation in older kids can be a little bit trickier. They don't always want to be motivated to do the things we want them to do. Words of encouragement sometimes aren't enough to make them try something new. In this and the next few chapters, I'll try to help demystify motivation by talking in depth about how motivation can be strongly impacted by a child's ability, the pleasure a child takes in doing things, and whether the child has developed any competence through practicing. Each one of these concepts—*aptitude*, *pleasure*, and *practice*—will be explored in depth in the next few chapters. For now, I'm going to give you some examples of how these concepts were important in lives of kids that I've known. Let's start with Bradley.

Before Bradley, whom you met in Chapter 1, was an unmotivated high school student, he was an adorable toddler who was cherished by his parents. He became a happy kindergartner and then an elementary school student who impressed adults with his knowledge of baseball statistics. His parents described him as "the most lovable child." Maybe he had difficulty getting himself dressed in the morning, or getting his homework done, or turning off the video game when it was time for dinner, but he wouldn't have been described as an unmotivated seven-year-old. Yet his parents would have said there was *something*. When I asked them when Bradley started not caring about much of anything, they couldn't pinpoint a day or a particular incident.

"It just sort of happened," his dad said.

"Yeah," said his mom. "Things just slowly got worse. I mean, he had trouble in school, but we could always blame it on something else. He was diagnosed with ADHD in second grade and had a great teacher who said she'd helped lots of students like him, but then she went on maternity leave in December, and she never came back. Bradley had substitute teachers for the rest of the year. That put him behind for third grade. Then in fourth grade we tried medication, and it took us a long time until we found something that worked. And then all of a sudden, he was in middle school, and then . . . I don't know. It seemed like he just disappeared."

"It was like yesterday that we were playing catch in the backyard," his dad continued. "He was happy. Now, it seems like he hates everything."

When I met with Bradley, I was pleasantly surprised to find out that he didn't actually hate everything. He liked his friends. He liked video games. He liked his bio teacher, even though he was late to class half the time and didn't do most of the homework. He liked working at Whole Foods after school and on the weekends. He even liked his parents and older brother and sister.

If you're thinking your child doesn't seem to like anything, is it possible that she just doesn't like what you expected?

When I asked him to describe why he thought he had ended up in my office, he described it this way: "My parents don't like it that I'm a slacker, but I'm okay. I just don't care about getting A's. What do I need geometry for? I don't care about going to college. I'd rather my parents gave me money and let me travel for a year until I figured out what I wanted to do. That would be a better use of their money. They want me to be someone that I'm not—like my brother and sister. I'm not them."

Bradley's description wasn't exactly filled with insight, and there was more than a little entitlement, but it gave me a place to start. Some of this data was easy for his parents to understand, and some was more difficult. But it was *all there*. Let's dissect this in more detail.

Bradley told me *he was basically "okay"*—after a more thorough evaluation, I was able to determine that while he still had symptoms of ADHD, he didn't meet criteria for a more significant mental health issue. He was clear that he didn't want to go to college, although I didn't see anything, like an untreated learning disability, that would prevent him from going if he changed his mind. He likely *was* different from his parents' other children. Perhaps that was a source of disappointment for them, or perhaps they just didn't understand it. Solving this part of the problem required helping them understand who he was.

Are you expecting your child who couldn't care less to be a lot like you or your other kids?

Helping his parents understand him would also be a way into helping them understand whether, and potentially how, they were inadvertently contributing to Bradley's behaviors. Bradley was clear—and correct—in saying *they want me to be somebody I'm not. I'm not like my brother and sister.* What *did* Bradley's parents want him to be? What did it mean for them to have a child who was so different from their other children? Helping his parents articulate answers to these questions would be important. Often the answers to these questions are poignant, and nearly always they have something to do with parental anxiety for their child's future. Sometimes it's because a child reminds the parents of one of their own family members—a sibling, uncle, or cousin—who had a life filled with disappointments. Sometimes it's because they can't imagine adulthood without a road map—high school, college, well-paying job. This is true even for successful parents who never attended college. Sometimes it's their own insecurities at play. *What will we tell everyone if he doesn't go to college? Or quits the soccer team? Or joins the chess team instead of playing basketball? Or dresses in ways where people might make fun of him?*

But while Bradley was right about a lot of things, his ideas for the future weren't quite realistic. Most parents don't want to hand over the money they've saved for their child's college education for a year of travel. This is completely valid and wise. But for a lack of other options, that scenario was the best Bradley could imagine. Unfortunately, guidance counselors (particularly in high-achieving high schools where college attendance is an important statistic) don't often engage students or parents in thinking about options other than college. If they do, it's clear that any other option is less than ideal.

These kinds of conversations need to happen long before college. I've talked to many kids in elementary school who were already worried about college in fourth or fifth grade. I've had third graders tell me that they are going to MIT or Harvard. It's unlikely that would happen, not because they weren't capable of being remarkable students but because statistically, it's probably not in the cards. However, someone gave that child the idea that's what the end goal is. By eighth grade, that third grader realizes he's not that special. Instead of having a conversation about realistic goals for the future, the child starts to check out. Sometimes he stops trying to do well in school. Sometimes the parents blame the school. The parents might seek a diagnosis that explains what's going on—and sometimes there is one. Or it might be blamed on the peer group or a hundred different things. Rarely is there one factor. Even more rare is an understanding of the child's personality factors, a discussion of alternative paths to adulthood, and an understanding of what might help or get in the way of being successful.

Mateo's parents sounded very similar to Bradley's. They came to me for a consultation when Mateo was 20 years old, hoping I could write a letter that would allow him to go back to school. They described him this way: "Mateo is a really creative kid. He loved art and graphic design, and we thought Hampshire College was perfect for him. He could create his own major! Who wouldn't want that? But after his first semester, he was put on probation. The academic dean told us that if he took a few classes for credit at a local community college, they'd consider taking him back. He hasn't even filled out the application. Instead, he went to Nordstrom and applied for a job. They interviewed him two weeks ago and hired him for the men's department. He can't wait to start next week. That's when we decided to call you. I can't have him working at Nordstrom when he could be attending community college next month and earning credits to go back to college. I told him 'Do anything you want to do. If you want to be a painter or a sculptor, I will support that.' I mean, if he wants to be anything—an artist, owner of an art gallery, anything—I'm open to it."

What if the goal that seems so set in stone— college—is not quite right for your child, at least not right after high school?

Do you see what's happening here? Mateo's dad is saying "He can be anything," but it's not true. Mateo can be anything as long as he finishes college and then does something other than work in retail. In fact, their dream for Mateo was that he would become an artist, like Mateo's father had wanted to be. I pointed out to Mateo's parents that their son wasn't saying he was excited about being a painter or a sculptor. He wasn't even as interested in "art and graphic design" as his parents thought he was. I also pointed out that their son had never painted or sculpted other than the required assignments for the two art classes he took in high school. Sure, his art looked good, but so did everyone else's in the class. Mateo hadn't felt the need to create anything else. At least not yet. And even if he had, imagine the kind of pressure that is put on anyone when someone who loves them says, "Go paint and sculpt! I will support you!" Even if a person were really talented, the pressure to produce would be overwhelming. Not to mention, most artists struggle every day with their own judgments about their work. (The college issue is discussed in more depth in Chapter 8.)

These sorts of struggles are magnified in an adolescent who is on his way to becoming an adult. Mateo's father's goals, while seemingly open to anything, were anything but. He could support a child who was a struggling artist—or at least he could support the fantasy of this, though I doubt he'd be feeling the same after a few years of support—but he couldn't support a son who wanted, at this time in his life, to work and gain confidence and experience. Those desires didn't mean his son wouldn't be a sculptor or a painter, or anything else sometime in the future. They just meant that Mateo didn't want to do that now.

Although I've been using examples from adolescents, these sorts of judgments and scenarios begin much earlier. They're just more subtle. For example, there's Terrell, the fourth grader who wanted to take ballet but whose father wanted him to join the rowing team, even though Terrell hated the water and the cold. "But I want to be his coach. I love rowing. I was a Division I athlete," her father said to me, as if Terrell's interests should revolve around his father's. Then there is Ted, the 12-year-old who was buying and reselling expensive sneakers on eBay. He was making money, but his parents were upset that he wasn't interested in baseball anymore. "He's not interested in anything," they told me, while also saying that their son had made $600 in profit the month before on his sneaker business. "You can't make a living at that," they told me. I had to remind them that Ted had a better chance of making a living selling sneakers than playing baseball. I also had to point out that they were wrong about his not being interested in anything. He *was* interested—very interested—in something. It just wasn't something they wanted or expected.

> When there's a mismatch between your interests and abilities and your child's, something's gotta give.

When kids' interests and abilities don't match their parents', something's got to give. Oftentimes that "give" can result in a kid who doesn't seem to care much about anything. It can be very hard for parents to change their perspectives. It's even harder for kids to change, particularly when we're not just talking about dreams (which can change, although that often takes time), but also personality and temperament (which don't tend to change). What are the factors that lead to this inability to understand our children? What are the factors that impede kids' ability to maximize their potential? Are these factors internal or external? Knowing the answers to these questions can be the first step on the road to helping your child become the person he's meant to be.

Aptitude, Pleasure, and Practice: Why Kids Do the Things They Do

In the examples you've just read, I've focused a lot on parental expectations. That's because it's a convenient and easy place to start. Parents—and parenting practices—are a lot more similar than the kids they are parenting. Parents tend to make the same kinds of mistakes. When we're talking about kids who couldn't care less, the most common mistake is that parents' expectations were formed without having an accurate view of their child's interests. In other words, *parents don't—or can't—listen to their kid's desires.* And it's probably because their own expectations get in the way. In the absence of knowing what their child needs, parents fill the void with their own hopes and aspirations. Sometimes these are things they wished they'd done when they were younger. In the next few chapters, we are going to discuss how to understand your child's interests and abilities in much more detail. Some kids are really easy "reads." You know exactly what they love. You might have a child who was born loving books and who is happy as long as she is reading. You might have a child who loves playing baseball and her passion for the game helps her stay interested in nearly every other facet of life. But this book isn't about those kids—the ones who tell you by their words and behaviors what sustains them. It's about the kid who never had a passion for much of anything, at least not for more than a few months or a season. They're kids who are hard to read and who tend to wilt under the pressure of parental expectations. That being said, I've worked with quite a number of kids who had an early passion for a sport or a certain activity, but who had an injury or major stressor in middle or high school. Deprived of participating in the thing they loved the most, they began to lose interest in everything and seemed like they didn't care about much of anything. During the pandemic, when lots of kids weren't able to do the things they loved doing, many kids seemed to look more and more like Bradley.

Yes, any child is at risk for just not caring, and there are at least three essential things parents have to consider in understanding why. I refer to these three things as the Parenting APP: *aptitude* (the natural ability we have to do something), *pleasure* (the enjoyment we get from doing something we love doing), and *practice* (doing something again and again for the purpose of improving or mastering it). As you can see from the diagram below, these three things overlap but are not at all the same. Of course, these aren't the only three things that underlie motivation. Life happens. Changes in the family or school can interfere with having the time or ability to practice. Losses can affect the pleasure we typically get from doing things we typically enjoy doing. Different kids react in different ways (see Chapter 6 for more information about how to take into account your child's unique qualities). All of these are important factors to consider, but without understanding the importance of pleasure, practice, and aptitude, it can be really hard to figure out how to get back on track after a setback, be flexible when things need to change, or even how to get on track in the first place.

WHERE DOES YOUR CHILD SHOW STRENGTHS AND WEAKNESSES?

Intervening with kids who couldn't care less depends on helping your child function in the area of "personal strength" instead of the area of "personal weakness." It means being attuned to their aptitudes, what they spend their time doing (what I refer to as "practice"), and what seems to make them happy ("pleasure").

Parenting APP Venn Diagram

Look at the three things that constitute a strength. All three of these usually are present in some way before we can call something a "strength." For example, we can have an aptitude for playing the piano, but if we don't get much pleasure from it and we never practice it, it's never going to be a strength. On the other hand, while these three things look equally weighted in the Venn diagram, even if two of the three of these are present, there might be enough to call it a strength. Bethany was a fifth grader with dyslexia who loved reading. Because of her learning disability, her natural *aptitude* for reading was compromised by her difficulties with phonics. However, she enjoyed books, had a superior vocabulary, and frequently *practiced* the skills she learned in reading tutoring. Her aptitude was supported by tutoring and exposing her to books to the point where she found *pleasure* in hearing and eventually reading stories. This led her to want to spend time reading (practicing her skills). Despite her learning disability in reading, reading became a strength for her. It's important to note that a little bit of aptitude can go a long way when nurtured by the environment.

Another child with dyslexia—especially one who doesn't have the appropriate supports—may find reading a significant weakness, given a vulnerable reading *aptitude*, low *pleasure* because he hasn't been given the tools to be successful, and a lack of a desire to *practice* because reading is difficult (we don't tend to practice things that we don't really know how to do).

Identifying strengths and weaknesses in your child is important because conflicts in this area can cause kids to not care and parents to care too much. In other words, the more the child withdraws, the more this can become an issue for the parent. Parents are supposed to care *a lot* about their kids' performance, but they shouldn't be more invested in the child's achievements (care *too much*) than the child is. That is a setup for conflict that can then progress to a child who doesn't care. In Chapter 3, I'll give you a much more detailed explanation of the importance of understanding a child's strengths, but briefly—if you're wondering how you'd even know if your child has a strength, look for things your child *tends to naturally do well*, *enjoys doing*, and *frequently chooses to do*. If you find your child enjoys something and does it frequently, but she doesn't display a natural talent for it, you can support her talents through enrichment activities and giving her space to practice. For example, if your child loves to draw and does it all of the time, but doesn't display much talent beyond drawing horses, you can enroll him in an art class and make sure he has lots of art materials on hand to explore his interest in this area.

Kids' strengths are typically things they do well naturally, enjoy, and choose to do frequently.

Weaknesses are typically things kids struggle to do well. They often seem unhappy when they are doing them, and when given a choice would rather do anything else. Kids don't have a choice when asked to practice some things that are difficult for them. They have to practice reading and learn their multiplication facts, whether they like it or not. That's part of life, but it's generally not a great idea to force kids to be experts in things that are difficult for them and that they don't need to know or do.

Other than skills they have to learn and practice, like reading, it's best not to try to force kids to become experts in what they find difficult and don't need.

For example, Jimmy hated math. It was a tough subject for him, but his parents felt it was important for him to take Kumon Math after school. For those of you not familiar with the fast-growing chain called Kumon Math, it's an afterschool enrichment program that is pencil-and-worksheet based. It's become so popular in certain areas that parents are afraid their kids will be at a disadvantage if they don't enroll them in it. There are other math tutoring companies, and they can be great for kids who love math. And I don't mean to pick on math. There's a seemingly unlimited number of examples that you could substitute for "math enrichment," ranging from gymnastics to soccer to Suzuki violin to creative writing.

While Jimmy didn't enjoy math at school, he was passing the subject with a B/C average without any assistance. But his parents wanted him to excel in math. They were both engineers and felt math was the foundation for almost any job they could imagine Jimmy having in the future. Jimmy despised his Saturday morning classes. He never wanted to go, and he felt bad about himself when he did, referring to himself as "stupid" in math. Enrichment math classes were a bad choice for Jimmy. On the other hand, his sister Roshanda loved math and had quite an aptitude for it. Math class was the highlight of her week, even when it occurred at 9:00 A.M. on Saturday. Math was clearly a strength for her, and this extracurricular activity was perfectly suited for her APPs.

I am often asked whether a child should continue to take music lessons or continue playing a team sport. While I encourage kids to finish a season or a semester, there isn't much good in forcing kids to remain in a sport or extracurricular activity that is difficult for them. Parents can also be frustrated when the child exhibits an aptitude for something but doesn't want to practice. Take Terrell from earlier in the chapter. His dad wanted him to join crew and said he had an aptitude. But Terrell didn't enjoy his time on the water, and he never chose to spend time on boats of any kind. I encouraged Terrell's dad to talk to him about it, by stating the obvious: "You've got some talent in crew, but I see that you're not enjoying it and haven't for quite some time. Why do you think that is?" In Terrell's case, it was because he didn't like spending his free time being cold on the water at the crack of dawn. He also didn't like the competitive aspects of rowing. "It's not my thing," he said to his dad. "It's not fun for me. You like it, but I don't." If he had said, "I hate my coach" or "I don't feel confident enough in my skills as a rower," I'd suggest trying to fix whatever was getting in his way. But the problems he was identifying were more about the activity itself, and it was unlikely anything was going to change. I suggested helping him find other places where he could excel, like ballet, which Terrell was already interested in.

"But What Do I Do Today, Doc?"

"But what do we do today, Doc?" Bradley's dad asked me. After meeting with Bradley individually, I scheduled an appointment with his parents to review what we'd discussed. I told them there would be many pieces to this puzzle and we'd take them one at a time. Setting mutual goals (something discussed in detail in Part III of this book) was a necessity and the key to motivating Bradley and decreasing parental anxiety. But goals can't be set until you understand what you desire to accomplish. At the same time, parents of kids like Bradley want answers *now*. I can't blame them. Unfortunately, there are no quick solutions. I realize this is not the answer you're wanting to hear, and I dearly wish I could give you a simple phrase or behavioral checklist that would get your child motivated. It's going to take some time to sort out—use this piece of knowledge to take some pressure off you and your child.

However, this doesn't mean there is nothing that you can immediately do. What you can do today—right now—is think about your child and where APP intersects for him. If you really don't know—or need help sorting this out—keep reading. Bradley's parents weren't sure either when I drew a Venn diagram and asked them to fill in the areas that applied to Bradley. In the circle labeled "aptitude," they wrote, "good with people," "good vocabulary" (relabeled from what Bradley's dad originally wrote, "can talk a good game"), "caring for others," "shows up for work on time when he likes the job," "writing, when he sits down to do it." Under "practice," they wrote, "working at Whole Foods," "playing video games," "reading graphic novels," and "hanging out with friends." And under "pleasure" they wrote, "working at a job that he knows he can do well," "reading," "playing video games," "being there for his friends," "spending time with his grandparents," and "taking care of animals." (See Bradley's Venn diagram on the facing page.) Until forced to write these things down, they hadn't realized that there were things that Bradley liked to do and was good at doing. While their other two children, who were focused on academic success, liked visiting their grandparents, Bradley loved being with them. Yes, he was a kid who seemed like he couldn't care less to his parents and siblings, but he got a lot of pleasure from helping others in ways that his achievement-oriented siblings did not. He hadn't gotten much reinforcement for those skills, but in reality, his strengths are much more rare than great grades on math tests. Although I hadn't yet given his parents any specific strategies on how to fix the difficulties in their lives, they left this appointment with a new perspective and a desire to better understand the problem. They also

Bradley's Venn Diagram

Aptitude

Can talk a good game
Good vocabulary

Good with people

Caring for others

Shows up for work on time
when he likes the job

Writing, when he sits
down to do it

Pleasure

Reading

Playing video games

Working at a job that
he knows he can do well

Being there for his friends

Spending time with
his grandparents

Taking care
of animals

Strength

Practice

Working at Whole Foods

Playing video games

Hanging out with friends

Reading graphic novels

had begun to grapple with the idea that Bradley's strengths might not lead to a direct path to college.

> *Identifying your child's strengths can uncover some rare qualities you haven't noticed.*

Wrestling with these issues might help you too, and the next three chapters will give you a better understanding of why they are key in understanding and changing the dynamic for a child who couldn't care less. It can lead you to feel less hopeless and more open to the idea that change is possible for your child as well as for you.

THINK, TALK, DO

What to Think About

- Think about your own personal strengths and weaknesses. How do they map onto the areas of aptitude, pleasure, and practice? Are there some things that are considered strengths that don't give you much pleasure? Why not? Thinking about these issues in your own life can be very helpful when thinking about them in the life of your child.

- What do you expect for your child's future?

- How did you form your expectations of your child's future?
  - What has your child explicitly told you about what they want in the future?

What to Talk About

- Open up a discussion with your child, focusing on the areas of aptitude, pleasure, and practice. Some questions you might ask include:
  - What are the sorts of things do you think you're good at doing?
  - What kinds of things make you the happiest? The most frustrated? What things make you want to try harder to do better?
  - What do you like doing? What are your favorite ways to spend your time? What do you like the least?

- You might already have an idea of your child's favorite real-life or fantasy heroes. If you don't, ask him who they are. Talk about real-life people they admire, both friends and family. Good follow-up questions include:
  - Why do like them? Do you want to be like them? Why?
  - Are there things you wish your heroes would do more of less of?
  - Are there things they do that you don't want to do?

- For younger kids, it's never too early to ask what they want to be when they grow up. For older kids, have lots of conversations about what they want to do after high school graduation. Don't just stop there. Ask "What would you need to make that transition successful?"

☑ What to Do

- Fill in an APP Venn diagram for both you and your child and the intersections. Have your child fill out one for herself. Is your version of your child the same as the one she drew? How is it different? Why do you think that is?

- For most of us, the intersection of these three things that comprise the APP don't typically look like a perfect Venn diagram. Sometimes you might find that aptitude plays a bigger part in identifying a strength and other times a strength is more the result of practice. Identify where these three areas are unequal and talk about why that might be a problem. Generate solutions to any problems when you can.

THREE

Aptitude

WHAT ARE YOUR
CHILD'S STRENGTHS?

About now, it's possible you are thinking "This is all nice advice, but truly the only thing my child seems to excel at is playing video games. You don't get it. He's not interested in *anything*. I'm not sure he has any strengths or aptitudes." If you're saying something along those lines, I'm here to tell you that your child definitely is good at something, but it might take a bit of digging and reflection to figure out what those strengths are. I find that parents who seek help for their child often fall on one of two dimensions—they see their child as having only strengths *or* they see their child as having almost no strengths. Either one of these extremes can be bad. A parent who labels their child as the "best" or "gifted" or "amazing" at almost anything can create a child who doesn't care when he realizes that he's not measuring up to an unrealistic notion of his potential.

Let's face it. No one is great at everything. We shouldn't put that burden on our children. If you're thinking you're the kind of parent who has done that, it's never too late to change. If your child is old enough to understand that you've done this, you can open a discussion. Parents begin using these phrases because they are completely in love with their child. Kids are miraculous creatures, and parents are incredulous about what their child can do. It can lead them to think everything their child has done is the best thing that has ever been done. If you're guilty of doing this, talk to them honestly about your motives. It's a positive way to describe why you might have put too much pressure on them or made them feel as if they were better than they knew they were at playing the piano or gymnastics.

The other extreme—and the one that is more common by the time kids who couldn't care less reach my office—is the child who has seemingly nothing going for him. I'm going to speak for my profession and take some of the blame for this. Psychology is mostly known for answering the question *"What's wrong with Imani?"* and not for helping to determine *"What's right with Imani?"* Parents understandably can have difficulty hearing me use terms like *ADHD* or *autism* when describing their children, but it can sometimes be even more difficult for them to leave my office when I don't have a clear answer to why their child is struggling—when there isn't a diagnosis that can be blamed as the cause. After all, parents come to me to find out how to fix a problem. Sometimes parents—and even kids—come to me with a ready-made label. It's not unusual anymore to get a referral from a parent that is something like "My teen thinks she has ADHD, so I'm calling you to see if she does." Or "If you could give my son the diagnosis of ADHD, he could get medication like his friend Bryce, and school would be so much easier for him and us too!"

The tendency to want to label or pathologize behavior has become pervasive, and parents become particularly desperate for a label when their child doesn't seem to care about much of anything. This need is based on the assumption that if we can remediate the weakness—if we can name the "problem" and the "solution"—the child will be happy. Labels are absolutely useful and necessary, but the absence of a label (or its symptoms) does not necessarily indicate the presence of mental health. In other words, there are plenty of unhappy, or at least less-than-satisfied, people who don't meet criteria for a mental health disorder. As I discuss later in this chapter, there are some real reasons, such as learning disabilities and processing speed, that cause kids to lose motivation. These issues need to be addressed, but they shouldn't be addressed without identifying a child's strengths. For some kids, just identifying their strengths could be considered a positive intervention.

Since we live in a culture where we are so used to going to experts to find out what's wrong, we might need some help in figuring out what is right.

Identifying Strengths

Positive psychology is an area of psychology that focuses on the science of better understanding what makes people happy and how to cultivate well-being. The father of positive psychology, Martin Seligman, viewed it as a response to the typical focus in psychology on mental illness, unusual behavior, and negative thinking. In the process of studying why people become pessimistic, he became fascinated with why some of us become resilient and optimistic. His research has led him to conclude that a fulfilled life means using our strengths daily in the major parts of our lives—for kids that means school, home, and social relationships.

Focusing on strengths is important because knowing one's areas of competence is associated with decreased stress and positive emotions. In therapeutic settings, using strengths as a way to understand oneself is associated with better outcomes. It can decrease symptoms of depression. Focusing on strengths can help kids meet developmental goals such as independence, relatedness, and competence. I mentioned *learned helplessness* in Chapter 1. It's the concept that when people constantly feel they have no control over their situation, they learn to give up rather than fight for control. In other words, they have learned to be helpless in situations where they might have been able to be actively finding and fighting for solutions.

Think about your child—or yourself. How much of your day is spent using strengths? For many kids, almost none of the school day allows them to revel in the things they do well. It is no wonder so many of them are unhappy.

It might seem counterintuitive to focus on the positive when your child usually appears

Kids who couldn't care less have often experienced too little focus on their strengths.

negative, but research has demonstrated that focusing on positive human development increases self-esteem, self-image, and overall well-being.

STEPS YOU CAN TAKE TO GET AT YOUR CHILD'S STRENGTHS

Identifying your child's strengths can take some effort, so here are some things to think about to get started.

If you don't know what your child is good at, ask someone who knows your child, "What are my child's strengths?" A great place to start is with teachers (if you're a teacher, see the sidebar below). Grandparents, aunts, uncles, neighbors, babysitters, and coaches are also terrific people to ask. When you go to your next parent–teacher conference, specifically ask about your child's strengths and tell the teacher that you're hoping to identify those areas so that you can make decisions about where to focus time in and out of school. Parent–teacher conferences are often about

How Can Teachers Help?

If you are a teacher reading this, you might be wondering what you can do to help identify kids' strengths. To be honest, none of us (including me) who work with children with challenges spend enough time thinking about strengths. It's not what we were trained to do, but we can do more (without taking too much of your already limited time). Take time to look through a child's record and note what others are saying about him (just as I've suggested parents do). Keep a happiness calendar for the class or have kids keep a happiness journal. It can be as simple as a daily sentence describing something that made them happy. Writing about what makes us happy is one of the easiest kinds of writing. It's also a great way to identify what we enjoy doing, which usually correlates strongly with what we are good at doing. Make sure you have some specific positive comments about a child's strengths when meeting with parents. If there are kids who really don't have many, let parents know that too. It's a sign that something isn't working at home or at school—or more importantly, within the child—and further evaluation or consultation with other professionals is needed.

weaknesses, and it's good to identify weaknesses too, but it's just as important to get insight into what your child does well. If you are the parent of a child who has learning or behavioral challenges, you might find yourself feeling discouraged after talking to teachers. *"Is there nothing my child does well?"* you might wonder. It's particularly important to identify strengths in these kids, as they are often the ones who grow into teens who don't care. There's no wonder why they might not care after years of people identifying only their weaknesses. I don't mean to characterize teachers as the culprits here—they're not. Oftentimes parents come to meetings already discouraged and wanting to discuss only their concerns. If you're a teacher reading this book, make sure parents leave every meeting able to articulate some of the wonderful things you see in their child. If there doesn't seem to be much to celebrate, make a decision to work with the child's parents to change that perception.

Reflect on when and where your child is happiest. Think about the instances where your child is exuberant about learning or doing something. Make sure you're distinguishing between being happy and being occupied. Kids are occupied when playing video games, but rarely are they truly happy. We're talking *happiness* here. If this is really hard for you—and even if it isn't—it might be great to keep a family journal about it. Write down when you see your child enthusiastic about something. Pay attention to their experiences. Ask them every day to name something that made them happy and write it on a calendar. You'll soon see some consistencies, and that is a good place to start. If you find that after a couple of weeks your child isn't showing signs of happiness anywhere on any day, it might be an indication you need to reach out for additional support (see Chapter 11 for more information about next steps if you're worried your child has little interest or pleasure in most things).

If your child has had previous testing, use the information from that assessment to get a better understanding of your child's strengths and weaknesses. If your child has been tested in the schools or privately, you have tangible data on your child's aptitudes/abilities. School testing often doesn't go into detail about strengths, as it's not the purpose of the evaluation (the purpose is to identify areas in need of support), but you can ask the evaluators to help you better understand what those strengths are and how they identified them. Private evaluations often identify at least a few strengths in the reports, but they are (and I am guilty of this myself) only a starting point. However, you can engage the evaluator in a discussion about what those aptitudes are, how they translate to academics and extracurriculars, and what you can do to nurture those natural abilities. If a private evaluator completed the assessment within the last few years, you can request to meet with them again. This may or may not be covered by insurance, but the additional information that a one-hour consultation can provide might be worth it. If the evaluation was done through the school, ask if there is someone at the school who can help you better understand the findings from your child's most recent evaluation. This is typically the school psychologist.

Look beyond the obvious extracurricular areas such as sports for areas of strength. I've seen many families completely dismayed because their child doesn't like sports. There is a lot more to life than sports. The *vast majority* of children *do not* play sports in college, and *even fewer* play sports after college. We spend a lot of time on something that kids don't tend to do after high school (and even after middle school for many). It's also important to point out that participation in sports as a youth doesn't necessarily translate to healthy living as an adult. That being said, sports are a wonderful way to learn about things other than the sport itself—but so is debate club, learning to play a musical instrument, and being in the school play. Beyond those activities, there are character traits—like empathy, the ability to persuade someone about your ideas, and responsibility—that can be strengths. These are skills that can be cultivated through tasks such as taking care of your neighbor's dog, working in retail, or working at a coffee shop. I see a lot of kids who seemingly don't care about much but are wonderful when working for others. That's often because their strengths lie in skills that are not what we think of as "talents." It's important to recognize and value those things. (If you want more information on what they might be, the Character Strengths Inventory at the end of the chapter lists the strengths identified in Seligman's research in positive psychology, with prompts to help you and your child identify them. There are also links to free tests you and your child can take online in Chapter 12.)

Listen to what people say who don't know your child very well. Sometimes good advice comes in the most unlikely of places; for instance, standing with other parents in the afterschool pickup line when they say, "Trudy is such a nice kid. She has been helping my Anita with her math homework every day during study hall." Or when a neighbor says, "Louisa has been taking my trash out for me on garbage day." Pay attention to those comments from these unexpected sources. Oftentimes parents brush these comments off ("Louisa? She doesn't clean up after herself at home!"), but they can be a source of meaningful information.

Finally, and especially if you're having trouble coming up with ideas, look at previous sources of data—e-mails from teachers, report cards. What are the words that are repeated for your child? You might be dismayed that there aren't enough good things that have been said, but looking through the contents of these correspondences can provide insight. Seeing a paper trail where there truly are no, or almost no, good things said about your child is cause for concern. Ask for a meeting with the teachers/administrators and tell them what you've found. Paper trails with little positive information can become self-fulfilling prophecies.

STRENGTHS VERSUS WEAKNESSES

The charts on pages 51 and 52–53 give some examples of what strengths and weaknesses generally look like. The first chart gives examples of academic strengths, while the second and third give examples of other areas. These are guides that you can use to begin reflecting on your own child's performance in various areas.

The "Child Interest Activity Checklist" from *Everyday Child Language Learning Tools* is a list of questions that can help parents determine a child's

ACADEMIC STRENGTHS		
	Reading and writing	**Math/logic**	**Specific subject (such as history, science, computer science)**

	Reading and writing	**Math/logic**	**Specific subject (such as history, science, computer science)**
Strength	Reads and writes at or above grade level Enjoys reading and writing Reads and writes during free time	At or above grade-level ability to manipulate numbers Likes to do math homework Manipulates numbers in everyday situations (adds up grocery bill totals, divides candies evenly)	At or above grade level in a specific subject Specifically expresses enjoyment about an academic subject Chooses to spend spare time working on projects related to the specific subject
Weakness	Struggles with grade-appropriate reading or writing skills Dislikes reading and writing Avoids reading and writing	Below grade-level ability to use numbers Avoids math work Dislikes math class and math homework	Below grade-level ability in a specific subject Avoids a specific subject Expresses specific dislike of an academic subject

interest. Though it's written for parents of preschoolers, many of the questions, such as *What "brings out the best" in your child?* or *What does your child work hard at doing?* can be answered for any age: *www.puckett.org/ECLL-Tools_3_child_int_act_cklist.pdf.* The questions help you think not just about aptitudes but also about the things that give your child pleasure (something I'll discuss in more detail in the next chapter).

What Is Aptitude?

The word *aptitude* is often used interchangeably with *ability* or *intellect,* but I like to think of aptitude as a potential ability. When you're trying to figure out why your child doesn't care about much of anything or why he seems unmotivated, you first need to figure out how capable he is of doing things, whether it's reaching an academic goal, playing a sport, or having a healthy social life. *Aptitude* relates to the capability of doing a certain task at a particular level. It's more about inborn potential, like an aptitude for music or becoming a pilot. It also includes things like interpersonal strengths and virtues, such as an aptitude for creativity, persistence, or social intelligence.

SOCIAL AND EMOTIONAL SKILLS

	Language	Emotional intelligence	Friendships	Executive functions/ organization
Strength	Large and expanding vocabulary Enjoys talking Initiates conversations	Accurately expresses own feelings and has insight into the feelings of others Likes to think about how other people think about or interpret events Spends time thinking about or discussing emotions and feelings with others	Maintains strong friendships over time Enjoys time with friends Dedicates spare time to social activities	Has age-appropriate ability to manage time and multiple tasks Enjoys organizing books, binders, or belongings Spends spare time planning or organizing
Weakness	Struggles to make themselves understood Dislikes talking around strangers, or at all Doesn't elaborate on answers ("yes" instead of "yes, because . . . ")	"Doesn't get" other people's feelings or misinterprets own emotions Dislikes expressing their feelings Avoids conversations about emotions	Has few friends Dislikes social interactions Avoids interacting with peers when possible	Struggles to manage time or multiple demands Hates organizing belongings or schoolwork Avoids spending time planning or organizing

SPECIFIC SKILLS			
	Music or art	**Athletics**	**Vocational skills**
Strength	Displays talent in art or music	Excels at athletic activities	Has a job, internship, or apprenticeship
	Expresses enjoyment or love for their artistic pursuits	Says they "love" their sport and smiles often when practicing	Expresses excitement about working and/or earning money for their labor
	Spends time practicing music or art without needing reminders	Goes to all practices and even practices their sport on their own time	Spends time preparing for work and is on time for their shifts/assignments
Weakness	Dislikes participating in these activities	Avoids going to games, participating—even when a team is doing well and the coach is great	Gets anxious about the prospect of having a job or working for other people. (Since this is a skill most kids have to eventually develop, it's important to think about this from the standpoint of finding the right kind of vocational experience that would decrease their anxiety or reluctance to work.)
	Struggles with the practical skills of artistry	Expresses dislike of specific aspects of the sport of the whole sport	
	Avoids practicing art or music	Struggles with athletic skills	

Ability is about having the skills to do something. For example, someone might have an aptitude for music. A child might be quite adept at singing and be able to play a few simple tunes by ear on the piano, but she wouldn't have the ability to play the piano until she developed the skills needed to master that task.

In coming up with the idea of the Parenting APP, it was easy to identify what I meant by pleasure and practice (more about those in the next two chapters), but more difficult to define the A—is it aptitude or is it ability? In reality it's a bit of a combination of the two, but aptitude is a better place to focus as it's less susceptible to environmental influences. This can also be confusing, though,

. . . . . .
Aptitude is an ability in the making.
. . . . . .

as intelligence and aptitude are often used interchangeably when they are not exactly the same. *Intelligence* is a general term that describes ability to reason, solve problems, think abstractly, and learn quickly.

HOW IS APTITUDE MEASURED?

In our culture, intelligence is measured by performance on an IQ test. IQ tests are a mixture of our aptitude for problem solving and the information we've acquired along the way (sometimes called *crystallized intelligence*). IQ is not a perfect measure of potential because crystallized abilities are in large part a result of our experiences and accumulated knowledge. IQ also includes things like working memory (our ability to remember small bits of information) and processing speed (our ability to do something simple in a given period of time), which aren't things most people consider "being smart." (For more on the limitations of IQ tests, see the sidebar on the facing page.) Despite some limitations, IQ tests are still useful measures of children's strengths and weaknesses as compared to their peers, though they don't include things like creativity, social intelligence, or musical ability.

If your child has had an IQ test, such as the *Wechsler Intelligence Scale for Children, Fifth Edition* (WISC-5; see the sidebar on page 56 for more information), it could be one source of data as you figure out his strengths and weaknesses. Most IQ tests have indices that measure broad areas of functioning such as language skills, nonverbal problem-solving skills, visual–spatial abilities, working memory, and processing speed. If your child scores highly in one or more of these areas, that area is likely a strength. For example, if a child scores at the 90th percentile on the Verbal Comprehension Index of the WISC, he's likely going to be good at tasks that require knowledge of vocabulary or verbal reasoning skills. A child who has high visual–spatial skills might be good at building with Legos, decorating a room, or imagining how things go together visually. Many tasks, from baking to biology, require good spatial reasoning

IQ tests can be useful as one source of information about your child's strengths and weaknesses but should not be the only source.

Limitations of IQ Tests

Though an IQ test can give some insight into a child's strengths and weaknesses, there are limitations that are particularly important to consider in a child who couldn't care less:

- They ignore creativity and the practical side of intelligence (things kids who couldn't care less often excel in).

- Many items are timed tests (something kids who couldn't care less tend to have difficulty with), and they wrongly equate intelligence with speed.

- The tests are culturally biased and don't take into account kids who "think outside the box" (something else kids who couldn't care less often do).

- Test scores are influenced by the child's level of motivation. Though the evaluator will try to minimize these effects, motivation can be more of an issue for kids who don't care.

- An IQ test doesn't assess a child's ability to acquire knowledge in the future. If a child scores poorly on an IQ test, teachers and parents might assume the child's future success is limited. This can lead a child to develop an attitude of not caring about much at all.

skills. One area of intelligence that tends to be weak in kids who couldn't care less is processing speed.

Other Factors That Affect Ability and Get in the Way of Caring More

PROCESSING SPEED

Many individual characteristics and life experiences can interfere with the ability to use our strengths. There's one characteristic in particular that I

The Wechsler Intelligence Scales

In spite of their limitations, IQ tests provide important information about a child's strengths and weaknesses in a few particular areas. The Wechsler Intelligence Scales—the *Wechsler Intelligence Scale for Children, Fifth Edition (WISC-5;* for children ages six to 16 years); *Wechsler Preschool and Primary Scale of Intelligence, Fourth Edition (WPPSI-IV;* for children ages two years, six months to seven years, 11 months); and *Wechsler Adult Intelligence Scale, Fourth Edition (WAIS-IV;* for individuals ages 16 years through adulthood)—are the most commonly used intelligence measures in North America. Various adaptations are used around the world. The Wechsler tests, and others like them, broadly measure two aspects of intelligence: verbal and nonverbal. *Verbal* tasks measure word knowledge, the ability to reason using words, and the ability to solve verbal problems. Nonverbal tests, sometimes referred to as *Nonverbal Reasoning, Perceptual Reasoning, Visual–Spatial Reasoning,* or *Fluid Reasoning,* reflect skills such as the ability to abstract information from designs and pictures, analyze patterns, solve visual puzzles, and build structures using blocks. Other aspects of cognition, such as *working memory* (the ability to hold information in your mind for a short period of time and use it while you're problem solving) and *processing speed* (the ability to quickly process visual information and the ability to make decisions rapidly), are also included on the Wechsler scales.

It's very common for kids who couldn't care less to have inconsistent performance on IQ tests. They may have strengths in some areas and weaknesses in another. This may cause them to be variable in their performances across different types of tasks, causing confusion in teachers and parents. That confusion might lead to calling a child "lazy" or saying things like "You were fine when we did this in class last week. What's wrong with you now?" rather than understanding that the change in the way the task was presented caused the child's weaknesses to become more pronounced. If your child has had a WISC or other IQ test in the past (even if it was a few years ago), it likely will provide some answers to questions such as *How quickly does my child process information? Is he good with words? Does he do better when information is presented visually?* and *What is his short-term memory like?*

think gets in the way of tapping into a child's strengths probably more than any other. A few years ago, I cowrote a book with Brian Willoughby on this topic called *Bright Kids Who Can't Keep Up*. The focus of the book was kids who processed simple information slowly. Most of those kids performed poorly on the Processing Speed Index on the WISC. Processing speed is the pace at which we take in information, make sense of it, and then generate a response. Some kids respond more slowly to information than others. That's normal. What's not normal is that we live in a world that requires and rewards quickness. This has presented a real challenge for kids with slower processing speed.

In addition to taking longer to do almost anything from homework to getting ready for school in the morning, kids with slower processing speed are more likely to have social difficulties (because social activities often require quick responses). They can be slower to come up with an answer to a question, leading to frustration on the part of the listener and speaker. Homework presents a particular challenge, as kids with slower processing speed not only take longer to finish homework, they also are more confused about what homework they are supposed to do (or how to do it) and are slow to get started on homework tasks. A high percentage of kids with slow processing speed have difficulties staying organized/planning, self-monitoring, getting started on tasks (not just homework), keeping track of belongings, inhibiting impulses, and shifting/transitioning. Many kids with slow processing speed meet criteria for a specific disorder such as ADHD, a learning disability, anxiety, or autism, but not all of them do.

> *Considering how tough it must be to hear "Hurry up!" all day, it's no surprise that kids with slow processing speed often become kids who couldn't care less.*

Since we published *Bright Kids Who Can't Keep Up*, I've noticed that many kids with slower processing—especially the ones who did not get appropriate treatment or accommodations—grow into kids who don't care. If you're wondering if your child is one of these, take a look at her WISC scores and see if the Processing Speed Index falls more than 15 or 20 points below the other indices or if it's low (below the 25th percentile). If so, this is a very important piece of the puzzle as to why your child might not seem to care much about anything. Imagine if you are always the last one done. Or it takes you longer to make a decision than the average person and no one waits for you. Or you live your life hearing many times *every single day* "Hurry up!" and "What's wrong with you?" and "Why does it always take you so long?" If you lived your life like this, you also might say, "I really don't care about any of this."

If you think this profile might describe your child but your child hasn't been evaluated, you can ask for an evaluation through your local school district. See Chapter 11 for more information about how to request an evaluation through your school system or through a private evaluator. For more information about processing speed, you don't necessarily need to buy *Bright Kids Who Can't Keep Up.* You can get it from your public library. I also have written and presented extensively on this topic—most of which is available for free on the internet.

Understanding whether slower processing speed is a contributing factor in your child's malaise is important. As more than one parent has said to me, "So what you're saying is that it's going to take my son longer to do things? I just need to expect it? I can deal with that." Understanding your child's challenges and empathizing with her can help thwart the tendency a child might have to not care.

While it might be hard to view a processing speed *deficit* as a *positive*, it really can be. You first need to acknowledge how the processing speed weakness makes life difficult. Is it mostly at school? At home? With friendships and social relationships? Once you've identified the problem areas, you need to make sure the correct supports—such as extra time on tests/ assignments—are in place to make your child's life easier. At the same time, you can come up with a list of things that are positive outcomes of taking more time. We spend our lives trying to slow down. Kids with slow processing speed do this naturally. Write down with your child what they like about themselves. And ask them why they think they're struggling.

One time a child said to me, "I think what's wrong with me is that I'm just a dreamer."

"I think you understand yourself very well," I said, "except for the fact that you think there is something wrong with being a dreamer. The world needs lots of dreamers. They're the people who imagine things that have never been imagined before! We need to find a way to make school easier for you so that you can have more time to dream. Having more time to dream and think might actually make lots of things easier for you."

You might be surprised by what your child comes up with when you ask him why he seems to take forever to get something done. It might be something you can turn into a positive—like dreaming—or it might be something that can be treated, like depression or anxiety. In either case, it's important to start with listening. Writing these things down—listing them as something to be celebrated or supported—is an important next step that helps a child see herself differently.

ADHD, LEARNING DISABILITIES, AND OTHER ISSUES

While I think that processing speed is one of the biggest contributors to not caring, there are other, more general issues that cause kids to just give up. These include ADHD; learning disabilities such as dyslexia, dyscalculia, or dysgraphia; autism spectrum disorder; depression; or anxiety. Sometimes psychosocial stressors (such as the loss of a parent, a family move, bullying) play a role. Other times seemingly good traits, such as perfectionism or high standards, are too much of a good thing. Any one of these issues is a stressor that can cause a chain of events that leads a kid to become unmotivated (more on stress can be found in Chapter 1). As I said above about slower pro-

All sorts of stressors can lead to a child's losing motivation.

cessing speed, make sure you identify the cause, determine how to remediate or accommodate the symptoms, and then see if any of these things can be seen as a positive.

Always Return to Strengths

Things like processing speed weaknesses and learning disabilities can interfere with a child's and parent's ability to see strengths.

Seligman has described a number of criteria that define a strength. Look at this checklist and ask yourself where and how much time your child spends in this "strength" zone as defined by Seligman:

- A feeling that "when I'm here, I'm the real me" (sometimes referred to as our "authentic selves")
- Showing a sense of excitement when doing an activity (your child can't wait to do the activity—drawing, playing basketball, writing)
- Doing something where there is a rapid learning curve, even as the activity gets more complicated (as things get more difficult, there's an acknowledgment that it's hard but also a desire to keep going)
- Time spent learning new ways to practice or use the strength (a parent might need to tell the child to stop doing the activity because it's time to go to bed)
- A desire to act in a way that honors the strength (the strength or activity becomes somewhat sacred to the child)
- A feeling of invigoration rather than exhaustion when using the strength (the child feels less tired after a great game rather than exhausted)
- Creating and pursuing opportunities to use the strengths (the child asks to do more activities—camps, afterschool opportunities)
- Intrinsic motivation (your child doesn't need to be reminded to do the activity)

How often does your child display any of the above in the course of a day? Or a week? Or a month? Probably not often. Many kids have only a few of these feelings in a typical week.

IDENTIFYING A CHILD'S HIDDEN STRENGTHS

We tend to think of strengths as "talents" or "abilities," and often they are, but I find that for kids who don't seem to care much about anything, their strengths frequently lie in their character. Seligman and his colleagues founded an organization called the Values in Action (VIA) Institute on Character. Their research indicated there are twenty-four character strengths, which can be divided into six categories:

- *Wisdom:* creativity, curiosity, judgment, love of learning, perspective
- *Courage:* bravery, perseverance, honesty, zest
- *Humanity:* love, kindness, social intelligence
- *Justice:* teamwork, fairness, leadership
- *Temperance:* forgiveness, humility, prudence, self-regulation
- *Transcendence:* appreciation of beauty and excellence, gratitude, hope, humor, spirituality

In the daily lives of school-age children, love of learning, curiosity, perseverance, teamwork, and self-regulation are the character strengths that are rewarded most frequently in school. Kids who excel in those traits spend lots of time feeling positive about themselves and their future. But what if your character strength is zest? Or the ability to forgive? Or humor? With the right teacher, any character strength can be seen as a positive. In the wrong setting, humility could be viewed as "not able to self-advocate." "Humor" could be seen as "disrupting the class." "Prudence" could be viewed as "anxiety," and "judgment" could be viewed as "an inability to see both sides." A child with "zest" might be labeled as "hyperactive," and even if a diagnosis of ADHD is appropriate, the idea of a zest for life is rarely part of the larger diagnostic picture.

A child who couldn't care less often has unsung heroes among strengths—those qualities that are not rewarded in school.

Years of not spending time in the "zone" of strengths, along with an adult or two who has identified a child's strength as a liability, can make a child lose interest in almost anything. Taking a close look at your child's strengths can help to balance out the negative labels with a more holistic portrait of himself. On pages 67–68 you will find a worksheet developed by the VIA Institute on Character that can be used as an exercise to rate the strengths of you and your family members. But you'll get even more information—a free computer printout plus tabulated results, by taking the *Signature Strengths Questionnaire* online: *www.viacharacter.org/character-strengths*. It's a free resource that anyone can use.

Using Strengths to Generate Solutions

After you've identified strengths, here are some activities you can use to move the needle from a focus on problematic behaviors to a focus on positive traits:

● *Talk about how each person's unique strengths can be used differently when solving problems.* For example, how might a person with the strength of "kindness" act when seeing a child being teased at school? What about a person with the strength of "humor"? What about when the situation is one of tension? How could humor be a positive attribute in that situation but not others?

Focusing on strengths has untapped power to build your child's motivation.

● *Talk to kids about what satisfies them.* What would they wish for if money and time were no obstacle? What are they good at doing? You can ask questions like these without taking any sort of formal test or questionnaire. Answers to these questions provide information about what a child perceives are his strengths and the meaning that he attaches to them.

● *If your child is artistic, have her draw a picture of herself at her best.* Writing a poem or making a video is another concrete way of expressing this.

Not all kids will respond to this, but if you've got a child whose strengths lie in creativity, this might be a better way to "discuss" this problem than talking about it in a conversation.

• *Families have character strengths and weaknesses too.* Spend some time thinking about the strengths that you as a family collectively possess. Do you possess strengths in love? Creativity? Humor? Do you collectively have a love of learning? Is spirituality important? As you're exploring these topics, be aware that it's frequently the case that not every person in the family shares what might be seen as a family strength. For example, Benny was a 12-year-old whose family appeared to possess a lot of social intelligence—everyone but Benny, that is. Benny felt like an outsider when his parents hosted BBQs at their house. Weekends spent camping with other families were torture for him. Benny possessed strengths in self-regulation and hope, so he didn't have the natural ability or see the need to express his feelings directly, but as he grew into adolescence, he began showing signs of being unmotivated. The rest of the family spent lots of their free time enjoying their strengths while he was miserable. Samantha, on the other hand, was a creative soul in a family whose love of learning meant they spent lots of time reading books and discussing ideas. Samantha preferred the bass guitar. While they all shared a common trait of *wisdom*, Samantha often felt like an outsider in her own family. This situation is very common for kids who seem unmotivated. Do some thinking as to whether something like this might underlie the behaviors your child is displaying.

Kids who spend too little time in their strength zone typically spend too little time experiencing pleasure. And as you'll find out in the next chapter, experiencing pleasure is key to helping kids *to care*—and a lack of it is nearly always one of the reasons kids learn to *not to care*.

• *Think about ways and situations where a lack of strength might be a challenge.* Are there areas in your family where no one has a strength? If so, think about how you can build up the strengths that aren't there. Or perhaps there's a strength lacking in most but not all of the family members. For example, if a number of people in the family lack social and emotional intelligence, have them learn how others make and maintain connections from the family member(s) who have strong emotional connections.

The Parenting APP

In the last chapter, I presented Bradley's APP—a diagram that showed where his aptitudes, pleasures, and practices intersected. Now that we've taken a deeper dive into the concept of aptitudes, I'd like you to spend some time thinking about your child's particular aptitudes. The diagram on the facing page is provided as a visual guide. The other two parts of the diagram are empty for now, but will become clearer in the next two chapters.

THINK, TALK, DO

 What to Think About

- When and where is your child happiest?

- Not sure about the answer to the previous question? Look at things that other people have said about your child—e-mails from teachers and coaches, report cards—to see what strengths and weaknesses your child demonstrates.

  - If your child has had neuropsychological testing done, look specifically at that report to see if there were areas identified as strengths.

- I've found that slower processing speed is a factor in a high number of kids who couldn't care less. If this is part of your child's natural profile, spend some time considering the role it might play in their motivation. If you're not sure, talk to the person who evaluated your child to get a better understanding of this issue.

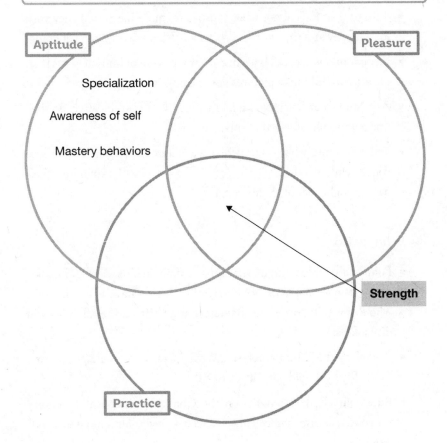

Aptitude in the Parenting APP Venn Diagram

Aptitude

Pleasure

Specialization

Awareness of self

Mastery behaviors

Strength

Practice

- How much time does your child spend in their "strength" zone? Keep track of this over the course of a week.

- What are the ways and situations where your child's lack of a strength is a challenge?

- Spend some time thinking about the strengths that your family collectively possesses.

What to Talk About

- Talk to your kids about what satisfies them. What would they wish for if money and time were no obstacle? What are they good at doing?

- If your child is artistic, have him draw a picture of himself at his best. Have your child take pictures doing things he loves doing.

- Ask your child, "Which adults in your life 'get' you? What do they understand about you that others don't?"

- Tell your child what other people say about her. "Your teacher says you're really good at _____" as a way of expanding their own thoughts about their strengths.

What to Do

- Point out people's unique strengths in daily life, movies, and books. Make it a regular part of your family's life to have a movie night where you talk about the characters and their natural abilities and difficulties.

- Complete the Child Interest Activity Checklist: *www.puckett.org/ ECLLTools_3_child_int_act_cklist.pdf*

- Rate your child's strengths on the Character Strengths Inventory (or go to *www.viacharacter.org/character-strengths* for a more in-depth look).

Character Strengths Inventory

Think about who you are as a person. Indicate whether each strength is mostly like you, sometimes like you, or not often like you. Realize that people have different strengths and that you can choose to build new strengths throughout your life.

Strength	Description	Mostly like me	Some-times like me	Not often like me
Creativity	I like to think of new and better ways of doing things.			
Curiosity	I am always asking questions and love to discover new things.			
Judgment	I look at all sides of an issue to come up with the right answer.			
Love of learning	I love to learn new things.			
Wisdom	I am considered wise because I evaluate things from different perspectives.			
Bravery	I speak up for what is right, even if others do not agree with me.			
Perseverance	I finish what I start, even if it becomes difficult.			
Honesty	I speak the truth and I take responsibility for my feelings and behaviors.			
Zest	I live life as an adventure filled with excitement and energy.			
Love	I value the close relationships I have with others.			
Kindness	I enjoy helping others, even if I do not know them well.			
Social intelligence	I pay attention to the motives and feelings of others.			

(continued)

Strength	Description	Mostly like me	Some-times like me	Not often like me
Teamwork	I always do my share and I work hard for the success of my group.			
Fairness	I treat all people in a fair and just manner.			
Leadership	I am good at providing leadership and direction when I am with a group of people.			
Forgiveness	I am willing to forgive someone who has done something wrong.			
Humility	I am humble and let my actions speak more than my words.			
Prudence	I am careful about what I do and strive not to do things I might later regret.			
Self-control	I pay attention and am always in control of what I do and say.			
Appreciation of beauty and excellence	I appreciate the beautiful and wonderful things in life.			
Gratitude	I pay attention to the good things that happen to me and express my thanks.			
Hope	I believe that good things are coming to me now.			
Humor	I like to laugh, smile, and see the good in all situations.			
Spirituality	I like to find meaning and a higher purpose in life.			

Looking over this list, what do you think are your five most important strengths?

Looking over this list, what are the strengths you would most like to develop?

FOUR

Pleasure

WHAT DOES YOUR CHILD ENJOY?

It's not enough to be naturally good at something; we also have to like doing it. Since there is a lot of overlap between aptitude and pleasure, much of what you read in Chapter 3 can help you determine whether your child finds something pleasurable. Kids who are naturally good at reading tend to grow up to be adults who read a lot. Same goes for kids who are naturally good at drawing, horseback riding, skiing, or robotics. But it's important to note that the difference between aptitude and pleasure is that pleasure implies they are doing those activities with enjoyment. How do you know when your child gets pleasure from activities that use a natural ability or aptitude? Typically, it's something they do a lot and feel great after having done it.

It *should* be pretty easy for us to figure out what makes us happy, but if the dozens of articles and books on how to find happiness are any indication, it's *not that easy*. "Do what makes you happy" is a popular piece of advice to graduates. What exactly does that mean? Therapy patients often spend a lot of time talking about their *wishes* and their *desires*—in other words, the things that would make them happy but for some reason have not yet been attained. Yes, we adults aren't very good at identifying what makes us happy. It's no wonder kids aren't either. It's easy for kids to figure out what is boring; it's much more difficult to figure out what might bring them joy.

If you think the only thing that makes your child happy is video games,

I'm going to tell you that's probably incorrect. Things like video games and Instagram and TikTok are placeholders that at best keep us occupied and entertained and at worst keep us numbed. People who spend a lot of time tweeting aren't doing it because it brings them a significant amount of pleasure. Yes, perhaps, making a TikTok video is fun for your child, particularly when done with friends. Some young people even get pleasure out of having a big social media presence. But for most kids, social media and screens merely occupy them when they can't think of anything else to do.

It's unlikely that video games are the only thing that make your child happy. In fact, they probably don't make your child happy but merely fill time.

In my clinical practice, I have new families fill out a form that asks the parents all sorts of questions about their child's developmental and medical histories and academic progress. I also ask a few open-ended questions, such as "What do you hope to get out of the evaluation?" One of the questions— "What do you hope your child will be?"—can be interpreted in any number of ways. Nearly all parents answer the same way: "Happy," they say. "I want my child to be happy." But, when I ask their children "What makes you happy?" many kids can't come up with much of anything. Despite parents wanting the ultimate goal to be "happiness," little time is spent cultivating it in their child or the family as a whole. And despite Western culture valuing the pursuit of happiness, happiness has only recently been a major area of research in psychology. Very little of that research has looked at the development of happiness in children. This might be because there is a perception from adults that kids are *naturally* happy because they're not dealing with the demands of adulthood. But a quick look at recent statistics on childhood depression and anxiety would indicate that is not the case.

To help your child figure out the things that bring her pleasure, you might need to listen really carefully. Hints might come out indirectly and sometimes in the form of envy or curiosity. For example, a child might be interested in the fact that another student is going on a study-abroad trip, going off to theater camp, working at the grocery store, taking up a new sport that few people play, like curling or fencing, or has won an award for something that your child might wish she could do. These are moments when you can help your child disentangle her feelings about why she is curious about the friend. Ask questions such as "Would you want to do that too?" and "What appeals to you about it?" It's possible it's something your child would *never* want to do, and that is meaningful information too. Listen closely to what sets off your child's small "beeps" of interest and use it as a starting point for more meaningful discussions.

Kids who couldn't care less tend to be kids who seem unhappy most of the time—they lack a sense of pleasure in almost anything. It's the number-one thing parents say to me when I have a child in my office who seems to not care about anything—"Nothing seems to make him happy." For the most part, professionals deal with this by trying to find the right diagnosis or cause. "He's depressed," "anxious," "learning disabled," "a bad match for his school placement." Any of these might be true, and it's necessary to address the issue if it is, but rarely do we go much further in the process—helping a child find pleasure. We want to "make him less anxious"—which we should, but we don't take the next step, which is "Now that he's less anxious, what can he do that will bring him joy?" As I pointed out in Chapter 3, focusing on weaknesses as it relates to children's aptitudes lowers the possibility that we'll be able to identify their strengths. Similarly, focusing on obstacles to happiness (while important to know) can fall short because it doesn't go the extra mile in creating happiness.

The Universality of Pleasure

Many cultures do a better job than Americans do of understanding and incorporating pleasure into their lives. Countries around the world, like Italy, France, and Greece, find much more pleasure in, for example, the act of eating. Studies have indicated enjoying eating sets children up for an adulthood where they are more aware of pleasurable activities. French children experience a life where they expect to relish the food they are eating, rarely talk about what they are not supposed to eat, aren't shamed for eating things that are caloric, and, thus, don't feel guilty when they eat something they love. The result of this ability to be mindful and not judgmental while eating is that French children grow up to have lower rates of obesity and many other health issues related to their diets. Food is not something to deny oneself, as we do when we diet. Instead, it is something to be enjoyed and mindful of. When we are mindful of what we are eating, we eat less of it because our senses are engaged in the process of knowing when we are full. Eating in front of a screen—mindless eating—increases the possibility that we will overeat.

Marie-Anne Suizzo, an educational psychologist who studies cross-cultural parenting, found that French parents do not consider *pleasure* a dirty word. In fact, pleasure is something that children are encouraged to experience, as pleasure is the North Star that guides them in determining their desires and future actions.

French parents educate their children from a very early age in how to savor and appreciate tastes. Dr. Suizzo's research found that French families rarely spoke about the nutritional value of or reasons *why* a certain food should be eaten. Instead, the focus was on the sensory experience of the food. And the education of "taste" didn't stop with the child's palate. It was about awakening all of the senses and the emotions. French parents tended to place more importance on what they called "stimulating practices"— things such as reading to children, playing music, or giving massages—than they did on things like teaching manners. Interestingly, Dr. Suizzo found that expectations for appropriate table manners were more easily enforced when children were expected to enjoy what they were eating and when the dinner conversation was along the lines of "This is delicious" instead of "Broccoli is good for you." The ultimate goal of stimulating children's senses in France was to help them understand what gives them pleasure.

A few years ago, I did a sabbatical in the Czech Republic, a culture not known for its healthy cuisine (though their obesity rate is still below that of the United States). I decided that since it was a once-in-a-lifetime opportunity, I wouldn't worry about what I was eating or drinking. I ate pastries with my coffee and meat with

> *Pleasure is our North Star, telling us what we desire and guiding our actions in the future.*

dumplings when I felt like it. They were delicious, and I enjoyed every bite. Some days I didn't feel like eating something caloric, but I never said no if I did. When I went out with friends, there was never a conversation about feeling bad about eating. In fact, the few times I reflexively said something about counting calories or feeling guilty that I had said yes to a serving of a dessert, my friends seemed very confused. If someone invited you to dinner and served a favorite dessert in this culture, it would be considered absolutely rude to say anything about why you shouldn't eat it. When you think of it, saying "Oh, I really shouldn't" when being presented with something delicious by someone who has spent time and energy buying or making something that will make you happy is a crazy response. And yet, these are the sorts of conversations kids in America hear every day. No wonder it's hard to figure out what makes us happy.

On my sabbatical, I found that, similar to the research on French parenting, taking pleasure in eating also led to heightened awareness of other senses. Thus, I was more aware that I'd enjoy taking a walk after eating a big meal, and I did it. In fact, I found that walking before or after eating made both of the experiences better, so I did more of both. Savoring a pastry at breakfast made me less likely to eat a large dinner. I was more aware of what satisfied me and thus what I needed to be satisfied. Mindfulness has been shown to be a good calorie counter, especially when the focus isn't on the calories but on the experience. On this "pleasure diet" I lost 10 pounds in six months (yes, you read it right—*lost*, not *gained*). There is something to be said for being aware of the things that make us happy. While there are many things that are better in the United States than in other places in the world, we have a lot to learn about pleasure and its relationship to child-rearing.

Activities That Focus on Product versus Process Can Sap Motivation

What does all of this talk about food have to do with your child who couldn't care less? Kids who don't care generally don't experience much pleasure in their lives. They often don't know what they want, and many haven't been happy since life shifted from play to school—when life shifted from process to product. Play can take many forms, but the essence of all play is pleasure. If it's not fun, it's not playing. Kids play with tangible things, like blocks and sand, and also with their minds through imaginative play. Most forms of play have no "product." Playing in a sandbox or finger painting isn't fun because you make something. It's fun because you play with something. Many kids who couldn't care less are described to me as having been wonderful babies and toddlers. As children they are often described as having a deep sense of empathy and understanding for others. They were the kinds of kids who excelled at playing. Some might have had difficulties controlling their impulses or getting out of the sandbox when recess was finished, but they typically had no trouble with the enjoyment aspect of play. They're the kids who enjoy reading when it's for pleasure (like graphic novels) but say they hate it when what they are reading is not something enjoyable for them. They tend to be the type of child who liked playing sports until sports became less about play and more about competition. As school and life became less about finger painting and more about worksheets and homework, they started to care less about things because there were fewer and fewer things to care about. They became apathetic—something I consider the opposite of pleasure.

Apathy: The Polar Opposite of Pleasure

Apathy is a lack of passion or enthusiasm for anything. It can affect a child's ability to be successful in school and social relationships. Everyone feels apathetic at times. Kids may become apathetic because they don't like certain teachers or subjects or for more complex reasons such as depression or an inability to grasp subject matter (see the sidebar on pages 76–77 for more on why kids become apathetic). During the COVID-19 pandemic, I heard from lots of parents who were anxious about their seemingly apathetic kids. Some of this situational apathy is normal, especially in the preteen and teenage years. Teens haven't yet found the emotional vocabulary to talk about what they don't like and why they don't like it, so instead of talking, they act like they don't care. They are hyperaware of what others think of them and sometimes will feign apathy because it's the cool thing to do. However, longer-term apathy, especially apathy with emotional detachment, isn't normal for teens.

Bruce was a 12-year-old who was described to me as a child with "no motivation to do, complete, or accomplish" anything. Even after 12 hours of sleep, he seemed to have little energy unless he was going out to meet with friends, where his energy seemed boundless. He wasn't interested in trying anything his parents suggested and tended to spend a lot of time alone, at least when he was at home. At the same time, he was quite animated around his peers. His teachers saw him as an engaged student. Although he rarely said a word at family dinners, when his uncle brought his young, hip, and very nice girlfriend, Miranda, to visit, Bruce spent hours talking to her about music and what they'd enjoyed watching on Netflix.

"He never talks to anyone, except you, Miranda," Bruce's parents would say. "Please come more often! You must have something special that we don't have."

What Miranda had was an interest in her possible future nephew, and that included no pressures or expectations. She just wanted to get to know him and find out what interested him. When he talked about a movie or a band she'd never heard of, she checked it out. Bruce responded to her interest in him and seemed like a normal teen around her, even if he didn't seem that way to anyone else.

While I was worried that Bruce could be on his way to being an apathetic kid who couldn't care less, I was less worried about him than I was about Tim. Tim had all of the same symptoms of apathy as Bruce and then some. His teachers were worried as he had become completely disengaged from the learning process. He was disinterested in social relationships of any kind, and after sleeping for 12 hours on a Saturday, he would get up, eat something, and go back to bed. Tim was more than apathetic. He seemed depressed.

Why Do Kids Become Apathetic?

Apathy in kids can show up for any number of reasons. Some of the most common reasons (especially in adolescence) are:

- *Pretending they don't care about something so that they can avoid feelings of failure.* This can be almost anything. Perhaps they had a bad season in basketball, or they are slow readers. They might tell you, "I don't like basketball anymore," or "Reading is dumb," because they fear they might not live up to someone's (sometimes it's just their own) expectations. Being seen as a kid who doesn't care is preferable to being seen as a kid who *can't do.*

- *Boredom.* Boredom is a word that can be overused, such as "Billy's bored in class, so that's why he can't pay attention." I'm not talking about that kind of boredom. I'm talking about the kind of boredom that happens as kids move into middle and high school and their interests change. Middle school is the age when kids begin to decide what they like and what they don't like. As they stop doing things they don't like (often because things they enjoyed doing require an expertise they aren't interested in—as is required in activities such as gymnastics, ice skating, ballet, and almost any competitive sport), they can have trouble finding good replacements. I find that high schools generally have a lot of things that kids can "plug into," but middle schools often don't have the same resources. In addition, kids are hypersensitive at this age about trying anything new. If you find this is a potential cause of your child's apathy, talk to the school about appropriate activities and ways your child can find new interests.

- *Your child might be rejecting your ideas of achievement.* Parents have dreams for their kids. It's wonderful when their dreams align with their child's. Oftentimes they don't. You might want your child to go to a certain college, achieve certain grades, play a certain sport. Your child might not want any of those things. Or he might prefer to think about these things and decide on these things on his own. A kid who doesn't care about playing soccer anymore might develop into a kid who doesn't care about anything. Trying to force your child's goals to align with yours won't generally work, and the way a child might tell you this is through her apathetic behavior.

■ *A child might want to show their independence.* The key task of adolescence is independence and differentiating oneself from parents. One way kids do this is by showing parents (through their "meh" behavior) that they aren't interested in life as usual.

When Is It More Than Apathy?

Tim's behavior worried me because his symptoms were chronic and getting worse. He was becoming more irritable and withdrawn and had few social contacts. Tim sounded depressed to me, and I referred him for a more comprehensive evaluation. Apathy that lasts for more than a couple of weeks at a time is often a sign of a more significant problem that needs to be evaluated. While many of the themes and recommendations apply, the treatment for depression needs to be more comprehensive than the suggestions found in this book.

Children and adolescents with depression typically have prolonged (more than two weeks at a time) bouts of sadness. They frequently have lost interest in activities and friends. However, some children—particularly teens like Tim—don't appear outwardly sad. Instead, they express their depressive symptoms through their irritable mood, so they may seem grouchy, cranky, touchy, or easily upset. In fact, irritability is one of the most common features of depression and is present in almost 80% of children with depression. (For more on depression, see the sidebar on page 78.)

Apathy that lasts for more than two weeks or gets worse may call for an evaluation for anxiety or depression.

Along with depression, what is thought to be apathy can be a symptom

What Are the Symptoms of Depression?

All children diagnosed with depression or a *major depressive disorder* experience either a depressed mood or a loss of interest or pleasure for at least a two-week period. In addition, they experience at least four of these other symptoms:

- Significant weight loss or weight gain or decrease or increase in appetite

- Insomnia (too little sleep) or hypersomnia (too much sleep)

- Overly active or agitated (very restless), or not active enough (can't get off the couch to do anything)

- Fatigue or loss of energy

- Feelings of worthlessness or guilt (*Why did I do that?*)

- Problems concentrating or a tendency toward indecisiveness

- Thoughts of death or suicide (with or without a specific plan)

of significant anxiety. Gabriella was a 14-year-old who, from an early age, had worried constantly about her schoolwork. In some ways, it made her a model student—until she entered high school, when the anxiety about being perfect, along with concerns that no one liked her and that she didn't fit in, became unbearable. Gabriella complained of chronic stomach problems, which were evaluated extensively by a pediatric gastroenterologist, but no problems were found. At night, she spent hours making sure her homework was done perfectly, but she was never satisfied. By the middle of her first year, she decided "school sucks" and stopped caring about almost anything. Had I not done a comprehensive evaluation, I would have thought that Gabriella was likely depressed, and while she had a touch of depression, her problems actually stemmed from an inability to manage her anxiety. (For more on anxiety, see the sidebar on the facing page.)

The good news about anxiety and depression as causes for not caring about much is that they can be treated. A treatment called *cognitive-behavioral therapy* (CBT) has been shown to be very effective in treating symptoms of depression and anxiety. A CBT approach helps children modify their thoughts and actions to reduce anxiety and improve their mood. CBT therapists provide problem-solving strategies and teach ways to cope with stress. Medication is also an option, as is support at school, such as meeting regularly with the guidance counselor or having a reduced workload to help manage stress. (See Chapter 11 for more information about how to get an appropriate evaluation for your child.)

Could My Child Be Anxious?

While many kids with anxiety are anything but apathetic (they can be "worry warts" who care too much), for some, apathy or not caring about anything can be a poor coping skill. Kids with anxiety worry about a lot of things, most of the time. They worry about *everything*—their family's health, whether the bus is going to be on time, how well they performed on a test, global warming, the homeless person they passed on the way home from school, the possibility of getting cancer, whether their friends "like them," the possibility of earthquakes or tornadoes—and the list can go on and on. Kids who couldn't care less and who have anxiety are struggling at two levels. They are anxious yet are working very hard at controlling their anxiety (which could be considered caring *too much* about everything) by looking like they care about nothing. Underneath it all is a child in a significant amount of pain.

Kids with anxiety experience physical symptoms along with their anxiety, such as headaches or stomachaches like Gabriella. Other physical symptoms can include a pounding heart, restlessness, trouble concentrating, irritability, sweaty palms, and trouble sleeping. Usually they're bothered by more than one symptom at a time, and the symptoms tend to change according to the situation. If your child seems to not care about anything and also is complaining about physical symptoms that have no medical basis, it's a good idea to have the child undergo a more thorough evaluation for an anxiety disorder.

The Biology of Not Caring: Willpower Isn't Enough to Make Someone Change

When we experience pleasure—that good, wonderful rush of emotions—we are actually experiencing the release of chemicals in our brains. These chemicals are called *neurotransmitters,* and their job is to send messages between brain cells. One of those chemicals is dopamine. People who experience depression can have too little dopamine as well as imbalances in other neurotransmitters. Rather than bore you with lots of details on the chemical structure of the brain, I will point out one important fact. Depression is a biological condition. It's not something we can think our way out of. People who are depressed don't lack willpower. Same goes for anxiety.

Recent research has shown that there is a biological basis for apathy. It's hard to know whether the feelings of apathy or the brain wiring came first, but the brains of people with apathy show fewer connections in the front part of their brains, making their brains less effective at processing information. Because of this inefficiency, it takes more effort and energy for a person with apathy to plan an action or turn a decision into an action.

If you've got a child who couldn't care less, it can seem *so simple.* All your child has to do is *care.* For some kids, it can be as simple as finding what they actually care about. But even that isn't just willpower—it's going to require reworking old habits and a lot of thinking and time. For those struggling with depression, anxiety, and chronic apathy, it's a biological problem that won't simply go away because of a desire to feel better. Luckily, the treatments for depression and anxiety (medication and therapy) lead to changes in the way the brain processes information. But again, all of this is going to take time, patience, and understanding.

Reversing apathy is more complicated than using willpower.

Beyond Biology: Why Some Kids Are Stuck in the Apathy Zone

Mihaly Csikszentmihalyi is a psychologist who has studied the pursuit of happiness and a concept he calls "flow"—that state where we are so happily engrossed in a task that nothing else seems to matter. We achieve flow when a task presents us with a high level of challenge and we have a high level of skill (ability) to perform the task. The lower the ability we have to use a skill, the more apathetic we are about the activity. The higher the ability level, the more relaxed we are, especially when we are not challenged. When an activity isn't challenging—when it's boring—*and* our skill level for it is low, we're disinterested about doing it. When the challenge level increases, it can lead to anxiety if we can't meet the challenge because our ability is low. If the task is somewhat challenging and our skill level is low, we might feel worried about getting it done. If it's somewhat challenging but our skill level is high, we feel a sense of control over the task. Finally, if the task is very challenging but we're very skilled, we can have that feeling of "flow"—we're prepared to do something that we can feel proud of accomplishing. Think of how it feels to hit a tennis ball in your racquet's "sweet spot" on a series of tough volleys or to whiz through a tough puzzle.

As you can possibly imagine, to achieve that state we need a high challenge and a high skill level that meets the challenge. Apathy is at the other end of this spectrum, and it occurs when we have a low skill level and a low challenge level. The perfect storm for apathy, according to this model, is a child who lacks the skills (maybe because of poor educational opportunities or a learning disability that has not been treated appropriately) who is put in an environment where he isn't challenged.

The opposite of apathy is flow—a state where your child is highly skilled in and challenged by the activity.

To move children from apathy to flow, two things need to happen—they need to feel successful in their ability to complete the tasks, and they need the environment to challenge them to think. I find that in practice those two things don't move together when kids who don't care are struggling. There will either be a push for the child to be less bored—"She needs to be challenged," the parents will say to the school. Or "He needs more reading support," the evaluator will argue. In the first scenario, a child might be advanced to an AP class without the skills needed to be successful, leading to more apathy. In the second scenario, the child gets more services in school to remediate the disability but isn't challenged by the rest of the curriculum because he spends much of his time in remedial work.

Getting this dynamic correct is difficult, and if this sounds familiar to you, you are not going to change it overnight. There are many other things you can do to help your child in the immediate future, but finding the right balance of challenging schoolwork and appropriate skill levels might require an evaluation by a professional. (See Chapter 11 for more information about this.)

SCREENS, SCHEDULES, AND SLEEP

There are some other things that get in the way of "flow" and that tend to make kids more apathetic. None of these three Ss will come as a surprise to you—too much time on *screens*, kids who are overly *scheduled*, and too little *sleep* are all things you've heard discussed in the media, at parent–teacher conferences, and at your neighborhood BBQs.

Screen Time. I could quote you statistics about how much time kids spend watching TV (an average of 28 hours a week) and how much time the American Academy of Pediatrics recommends they spend on all screen time (less than two hours a day for *all* screens) but that alone will not change your family's habits. It's just too hard to do. Take note of exactly how much time your child spends on screens. I want you to keep in mind that the time they spend on screens is passive, noncreative time that they could be spending on social interactions, abstract thinking, creativity, and play. There are some great books about how to tackle this problem (see Chapter 12), and limiting screen time is a good idea for *everyone*, not just kids. Spending too much time on screens is a cause of increasing apathy in our kids, but it's not the only cause, and in some cases it's a symptom. In other words, a child whose life is in the bottom left-hand corner of the "flow" chart is going to play more video games because it's the only place she feels good. Limiting her time playing video games isn't going to move her into a different area of that chart, unless other things—appropriate educational environment, a skill set that will meet the challenges—are put into place.

Schedules and Sleep. One of the biggest inhibitors of pleasure and joy is a child's schedule. Kids are overscheduled (more about that in the next chapter) and overtired, with a lack of sleep being the other thing that interferes with happiness and mood. Part of this problem is the world in which we live. Parents are afraid their kids will "miss out" on something. (It's not just kids who suffer from FOMO!) School days start before the sun rises, and afterschool activities last long into the night. Kids have little time to themselves. Young kids don't have time to play, and older kids don't have time to play with ideas. Next time your child says "I'm bored," do what my parent's generation did. Give them the option to do a chore or to "find something to do." Kids will find something. They'll pick up a book, sit in their room and imagine things, or spend time outside. If sleep is a big problem in your family, check out some of the resources we recommend at the end of this book. If you've got a child who is having difficulties managing screens, sleep, or schedules, you might find yourself yelling a lot of the time. At other times, when your child is managing a schedule or doing something other than spending time on a screen, you might find yourself praising even the smallest amount of effort. That well-intentioned inclination is not always in your child's best interest.

WHY PRAISE ISN'T ENOUGH

Our natural tendency when someone is struggling is to say "You're doing great" or to make them feel better about themselves by praising them. Sometimes this is related to our unrealistic expectations, and at other times we're just so relieved our child is doing anything other than playing Fortnite.

Remember Gabriella, the anxious girl you met earlier in this chapter? The first time I met with Gabriella and her mom, Gabriella's mom said, "I tell Gabriella all the time how wonderful she is. Why doesn't she feel better about herself?"

Gabriella's response was completely predictable: "I'm your daughter. Of course you're going to think I'm wonderful."

"But you are wonderful. Dr. Braaten, tell her she's an amazing kid. I know she could get into Harvard or some other great college. She's that smart!"

"You just don't understand," Gabriella replied before I could get a word in edgewise.

Both Gabriella and her mom were correct. Gabriella was a terrific kid *and* her mom didn't understand. She didn't understand Gabriella's struggles, and she also didn't understand how incorrectly praising kids can lead them to become apathetic and not care.

> *False or exaggerated praise, while well intended, can sap your child's motivation.*

This might seem counterintuitive—how can telling someone they're great be bad for them? But a wealth of studies done on this topic shows that the wrong kind of praise—one that praises intelligence, perfection, or talent—can do more harm than good. Being praised for their intelligence ("You're so smart!" "Look at those grades!" "You're brilliant!") tends to undermine children's confidence. Kids who get too much praise are less likely to take risks, are highly sensitive to failure, and are more likely to give up when faced with a challenge. I find the more a child is struggling, the more likely a parent is to use this type of praise, sometimes in an even more damaging way by pairing it with how he's failed to use his intelligence: "Brad is a gifted student. He's smarter than anyone in the family, but you wouldn't know it by looking at his grades."

Why can this type of praise be a bad thing? When kids are given this type of praise, they believe they are valued only for being intelligent, and it makes them not want to learn because they feel they should do well without any effort. The child feels she is being judged for the label and not for her actual capabilities. Like Gabriella, the child becomes risk-averse and doesn't want to be placed in a situation where she might be considered "dumb." She coped by starting to look like she couldn't care less about school, when in reality she cared a lot. I don't have data on this yet, but it's been my clinical experience that the majority of teens who don't care tend to have intellectual skills in at least one area (often more) that is above average.

But kids do want to be praised, and the way to do it is to praise their effort, their concentration, and their strategies. If they are acing their math class, use it as a discussion point as to whether they'd like to try a tougher class next year: "You seem to be working hard in Mr. Greene's class. I'm very proud of how you've managed the workload. How did you do it? Do you think you'd want to try a more challenging class next year, or does this feel right to you?"

Conversely, and this might hurt to hear, when your child clearly isn't the best at something, it's okay to say it. Heather was a sixth grader who decided to try out for the basketball team. She'd never played basketball before, but her best friend was on the team, and she wanted to do it too. By the middle of the season, Heather had yet to make a basket. Rather than tell her how good she was or complain that the coach didn't let her play enough, her dad said, "You're not as good at basketball as the other kids who've been playing on the team for the past few years. That's okay. I'm glad you decided to try it, and I admire your enthusiasm for practicing it even though it's hard. If it's something you want to get better at, I can spend some more time practicing with you. If it's not something you enjoy doing, you don't have to sign up for the team again. I'm just proud that you tried something new."

Increasing Pleasure

I hope that in addition to thinking about pleasure and apathy in this chapter, you've been able to take away a few things you can do to increase pleasure and decrease apathy. Some things, like changing the way you praise your child, can be done right away, while other things, like the right school environment, cannot. Nothing—*and I will repeatedly say this throughout the book*—not one *single* thing will make a difference on its own. Changing a little something here, gaining a greater understanding there, beginning a long-term plan for more challenging issues—together they will make a difference over time.

In addition, you can help your child be more aware of the pleasurable things in his life. One of the first things I would suggest is to take a look at how much pleasure is happening in your life. It's hard for kids to find pleasure when we ourselves make little time for it. Here are some other suggestions:

• *Make sure you have a household where self-sacrifice and hard work aren't the only things that are valued.* Don't get me wrong, these are great values, but in households where it's the only thing, kids often do one of two things—either they overvalue hard work and become overworked and anxious at a young age *or* they look at their unhappy and overworked parents and say, "Yeah, I'm not doing that." Also be aware of the tendency to overwork and overplay—where hard work is "rewarded" by intense periods of overeating or "relaxing" (letting go too much) to excess. That tendency is particularly difficult for the "apathetic" kids, who gravitate toward embracing the side of excess rather than hard work. Lives shouldn't be balanced at the extremes. It can cause some kids to have difficulty finding a middle ground that includes happiness.

• *Spend time with your child doing pleasurable things.* This is much easier when your child is younger and you can spend time reading to them, playing music, or giving them foot massages. Doing pleasurable things helps your child know what makes him happy. For older kids, it might mean dropping what you're doing when they say, "Mom, look at this *South Park* episode." Doing noncompetitive physical activities is also good—hiking, bike riding—or competitive activities with an emphasis on playing.

• *Try to have family dinners.* Having a daily meal together is a key way to infuse pleasure into a family system. First of all, if the earlier paragraphs about food weren't clear enough, I'm advocating that you make dinnertime a time of pleasure, with regard to food and conversation. While this can be a time to talk about important social issues, that might not be the best conversation for all of those at the table. Use family meals as a way to practice mindfulness. Eat together at the table. Avoid distractions such as phones and any other devices. Express gratitude in some way. Even if you can't do a family meal every night, making it a practice on the days you can might be an important element of helping your child become more aware of pleasurable experiences.

• *Cultivate gratitude.* Feeling gratitude is an essential skill that is associated with many positive psychological and health benefits, such as improved sleep, decreased aggression, reduced depression, and better self-esteem. Giving kids the exercise of saying something they are grateful for each day (perhaps at the family dinner table) helps build a sense of gratitude. Find

> *Cultivating pleasure is cultivating motivation.*

causes they are interested in and help them participate. Giving to others helps us appreciate our own lives more. Oftentimes, the things we are thankful are also things that give us pleasure.

The Parenting APP

So now that you have some knowledge about two aspects of the Parenting APP—*aptitude* and *pleasure* (see the diagram on the next page)—it's time to explore the third: *practice*. But before we get to that, here are some ideas about what to think about, what to talk about, and what to do.

THINK, TALK, DO

☀ What to Think About

- What brings you pleasure? If you're having trouble identifying it, start by thinking about what makes you grateful.

- After you've spent some time thinking about what gives you pleasure,

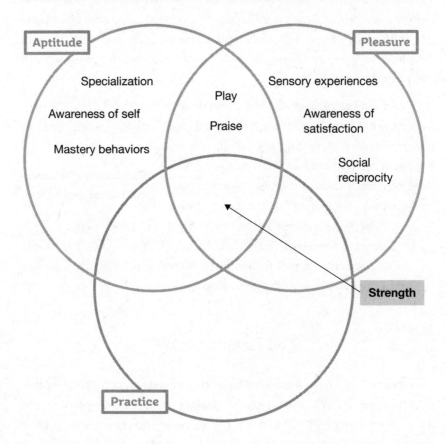

Aptitude and Pleasure in the Parenting APP Venn Diagram

Aptitude

Pleasure

Specialization

Play

Sensory experiences

Awareness of self

Praise

Awareness of satisfaction

Mastery behaviors

Social reciprocity

Strength

Practice

think about what brings your child pleasure and then think about the things that bring you pleasure together.

■ Don't forget to savor the good times. Take note of when your child experiences a sense of wonder or feeling of joy. Noting this together can strengthen their connection to what they enjoy doing (and possibly weaken their tendency toward apathy). If you can pair it with an acknowledgment of gratitude, even better.

What to Talk About

- When an activity or class ends, take time to reflect, and ask your child:
  - What did you like about this?
  - Did that feel too challenging or too easy?
  - What do you want to change about it next year?
- Ask your child:
  - What things are hard for you, but you like doing them anyway?
  - What do you look forward to?
  - What makes you feel excited?
  - If you could take one thing *off* your schedule, what would it be? If you could put one thing *on?*

What to Do

- Next time your child says "I'm bored," give them the option to do a chore or to "find something to do." If you can tolerate them complaining for long enough for them to actually find something else to do (this is not easily done), you might observe that they gravitate toward certain kinds of activities, like outdoor play or messing around on Dad's old bass guitar. Use this information as a way to help them set goals (more information about goal setting in Chapter 9).
- Track your child's time expenditure: How much time are they spending on screens? In activities? Sleeping? How much time is left over to *play* and *explore?*
- Spend time with your child doing pleasurable things.
- Have some family dinners on a regular basis (here is a great resource on the topic: *https://thefamilydinnerproject.org*).
- Practice gratitude.
- Notice when your child talks about another child's activities and ask questions such as "Would you want to do that too?" and "What appeals to you about it?"

FIVE

Practice

WHAT DOES YOUR CHILD PERSIST AT?

Practice is often thought of as a dirty word. It might bring up negative connotations of sixth-grade trombone lessons or math flash cards. But that's not actually what I'm talking about. I'm talking more about practice as *doing*—doing the things you can do well and that give you pleasure. For kids, it's about doing these things *independently*. To better understand this kind of practice, you'll need to spend some time observing how much time your child spends doing something without your having to nag him about it.

Practicing something like the piano doesn't just lead to learning how to play a tune. It also develops skills like discipline and time management. As children practice skills, they gain mastery, which creates competence. They learn how to *show up*—how to be reliable and consistent—which is an essential component in learning how to achieve goals. But the benefits don't stop there. Practicing a skill actually causes changes in brain structure. As we learn something, like riding a bike, our brain builds pathways between different areas of the brain. The coating on our brain cells that help these cells communicate with one another, the *myelin coating*, becomes thicker, which means our actions become more automatic and quicker. As you watch a child learn to ride a bike without training wheels, you're actually watching him build connections in his brain in real time.

Why is this important to kids who couldn't care less? Lots of apathetic kids spend little time practicing things they enjoy. This can lead to a cycle of low motivation, but it also leads to brains that are less wired to make connections that lead to better skills and increased overall motivation. Understanding the role of practice in your child's life is important for two reasons. First, practicing, whether it be math facts or piano scales, might be a source of strain in your relationship, and knowing when it's good and when it's unnecessary might relieve some familial stress. Second, a deeper understanding of the positive role of practicing can help you know how to use it to motivate and challenge your child to care more about things he once found enjoyable as well as help him find new pleasure in activities.

Practice: Where Aptitude and Pleasure Combine as a Desire to Do Something

While the word *practice* may sound like something we do that's hard, that's not most often the case. Practice is simply an activity we repeat regularly. This means that we all spend time practicing things every day. We practice cooking, making the bed, riding our exercise bike. Kids practice many tasks at school, from memorizing math tasks to learning to draw. Lots of practicing involves doing things we already know while we are only partly focused. This kind of practice, when it involves something like playing the same scales on the piano without thinking of them, is often not very fun, and it's not particularly effective. But there's another way to think about practicing, and it has to do with intentionality or deliberateness.

Deliberate practice is the opposite of the rote repetition that everyone hates.

Deliberate practice is a term that's become popular in psychology and education. It's the opposite of *rote repetition*—repeating a task over and over again until you learn it. Instead, deliberate practice is an intentional, purposeful approach to learning something new or getting better at a skill you've already learned. Here are some of the key ingredients of deliberate practice:

• *It focuses on the things that are hard.* It's not about doing one-minute math worksheets composed of multiplication facts. It's about tackling something that's more difficult—the problematic passage in a piano piece or a particular type of serve in tennis.

• *It requires concentration.* This means that social media, the phone, friends can't be nearby. It can help to talk to kids about this as being "their time" or "me time." Instead of telling them what they *can't* have, talk about it in terms of it being a wonderfully selfish time where they can learn something new.

• *Deliberate practice requires feedback.* This means that an adult needs to be around to help the child know where he has made mistakes. If a child is practicing long division, the teacher won't be there while the child is doing his homework but should be available the next day to review what went right and what didn't. As an aside, this is one of many reasons why too much homework isn't a good thing. Too many math problems for homework changes what could be a deliberate practice exercise (do two problems with intentionality) into one in which speed and rote skills are rewarded (do 10 problems and don't forget to bring it back completed tomorrow whether you truly understood it or not). More problems on a homework assignment mean that there are fewer opportunities for deep one-to-one feedback from the teacher. Instead, the feedback tends to just be a percentage correct on the homework assignment with a "See me" at the top of the page if the performance was less than stellar. No one wants to spot a "See me" on a homework assignment, and most kids who get a "See me after class" don't willingly go for extra help, in part because the opportunity for learning has passed by. Added to that are frequent feelings of shame (despite the often good intentions of the teacher).

• *It's not just a one-time thing.* Deliberate practice requires, well, *practice*, until you reach mastery. The difference is that it's goal-focused and meaningful. Kids might not always find it inherently enjoyable. That's okay. Encouraging children, pointing out how practice is making a difference, expressing confidence in the child's ability to succeed in solving problems, and designing activities/practice sessions that maximize their ability to be successful is key.

If you're a teacher, see the suggestions in the sidebar on page 94.

How Much Practice Is Really Necessary?

We tend to think that the most talented people in the arts and sports practiced hours every day as a child. The research has shown this is not the case. Instead, kids start out small and increase little by little over time. A study by Anders Ericsson and his colleagues found that expert violinists practiced no more than five hours a week in early childhood. However, by the time they were in their 20s they practiced 30 hours a week. Of course, by then it was their career and 30 hours a week was reasonable. Because deliberate practice takes a lot of concentration, kids don't need to do too much of it to make a difference. This applies especially to activities that tax the body, such as sports. There's an assumption that a child who shows talent for soccer will need daily, yearlong practice sessions. From my vantage point, this assumption can lead to problems. One specific group of kids I see who couldn't care less are the kids who were once thought of as sports stars at age eight but by 15 had sustained an injury or weren't good enough to make the travel team. Most were devastated by the loss, but some were relieved of the stress. Nearly all the kids who reached my office had lost a sense of purpose and sometimes their entire peer group. The idea that spending a lot of time practicing is a good thing can be a setup when something goes wrong. It's also a really boring and mundane way to spend a childhood.

So what is reasonable in terms of practicing skills? In the sidebar on pages 96–99, I provide some data-based guidelines as to what is appropriate for different ages with regard to practicing and homework. Much of the research

You might be surprised by how little homework should be assigned before high school.

Just for Teachers

While parents have to live with the child who practices, teachers of all kinds—classroom teachers, athletic coaches, music teachers, art teachers—are arguably the ones who are most often responsible for guiding children on *what* and *how* to practice. If you're a teacher, you're likely already using some of these suggestions naturally, but they're worth repeating, as these recommendations can help the child who is apathetic in the classroom.

- Wait until kids need more information to solve a problem before you give them the information. It helps them avoid becoming over-whelmed and also helps them think through the next step.

- Break down complex problems into smaller steps. If it's an algebra problem, make sure they know how to solve each step along the way.

- Kids don't respond well to practicing information in the same way over and over again. Mix things up.

- Kids should have had plenty of opportunities to practice applying problem-solving skills before they are tested on their ability to use those skills.

- Before you ask a child to practice something independently, make sure you have shown him how to do it. As many parents can attest, lots of homework assignments that are meant to practice skills that were learned in class don't come with a model or an example.

- Similarly, don't give students problems that are *too* hard or for which they *don't have the actual skills* needed to solve the problems you'd like them to practice. Practicing involves consciously doing something that is neither too easy (or already learned) nor too difficult (because it hasn't yet been learned).

- A little bit of practice over many days is much more effective than a lot of practice over just a few days.

on practice relates to reading, one of the most important skills to practice, as it is the foundation for all learning.

Things That Get in the Way of Practicing

If practicing is so good for kids, why don't they do more of it? And why is it that the kids who couldn't care less particularly hate practicing? The obvious reasons are that learning something new and practicing it regularly can sometimes be tedious. Or sometimes hard. And both can make a child want to stop practicing. There are many things that can distract a child from practicing—interesting things like social media and social relationships but also difficult things like family stressors, illnesses, and injuries. For kids who don't care, it can often be that they never experienced much success from practicing. They were asked to practice things they weren't ready to do yet. They didn't get appropriate feedback on their progress, so they didn't think anyone took an interest. A lot of practicing in elementary school involves practicing schoolwork, and if a child has a learning disability that went undiagnosed or untreated, a child can feel the whole idea of practicing is completely futile. "It didn't work, so why bother?" is often what they've learned. I've said this before, but if you suspect your child has a learning disability or attention problem, get more information. Attempting to practice something we don't understand or that we can't pay attention to is like asking someone who needs glasses to read the blackboard from the back of the room. No matter how hard they try, they cannot do it. It will lead to demoralization, demotivation, and a tendency to become apathetic and unmotivated.

Could your child have a learning disability? It's only natural for a child to be demoralized and demotivated by having to practice something that the child simply cannot do.

In addition to these issues, research has shown there are two things that get in the way of practicing—the wrong kind of motivation and too little time.

Developmental Timeline for Practicing and Homework

PRE-ELEMENTARY STUDENTS

■ Nearly any skill that a child acquires before first grade is done through deliberate practice—from walking to talking to learning how to tie shoes. There is little need to structure "practice sessions" as children naturally practice these things deliberately.

■ If you have a child who shows a particular talent or interest in something, such as art, sports, or music, keep it fun for now. Make sure the teacher or the coach understands early childhood development. Most kids this age, if given the time, space, and *no* pressure, will play around with their talent. Let them do it.

■ Even world-class violinists practiced fewer than five hours a week in early childhood. There likely isn't anything children at this age should be practicing more than three hours a week unless they are "playing" with the skill.

ELEMENTARY STUDENTS (GRADES K TO 5)

■ Early-elementary-school students (grades 1 to 3) benefit very little or not at all from homework, as there is no relationship between time spent on homework and academic achievement. For grades 3 to 5, the data is mixed but not very strong. Overall, kids this age do better with supervised, in-school practicing.

■ In terms of extracurriculars, this should be a time when kids are exposed to a wide range of experiences. When they begin a new activity, it should be one in which they express interest and then take it slowly. For example, if your child wants to play the violin, don't start by buying an instrument. It puts too much pressure on the child. At the same time, this is a good age to learn how to honor one's commitments. Practicing every day for 15 to 20 minutes will be important. If they've decided to learn karate, they need to go for the entire term. Let them know they can quit if they want, but not until after the term/season is over.

- Practicing phonics has been shown to be an effective way to increase reading skills in readers with and without learning disabilities. Oral reading is also something that is helpful to practice, as it leads to stronger reading performance later on.

- Practicing vocabulary through talking about words, reading books, and learning vocabulary lists from school has a very positive effect on later vocabulary.

- Drill-repetition-practice (times tables, spelling words) has been shown to be beneficial for students with learning disabilities across all age groups. Practicing these skills in fun, game-based ways makes the practicing much more deliberate.

MIDDLE SCHOOL STUDENTS (GRADES 6 TO 8)

- One to two hours of homework a night (but no more) for middle school students does show some benefits on learning.

- This is a good age to pick just one (at the most two) extracurricular activity to do at one time. Thirty minutes of deliberate practice at this age five to seven times a week can be enough for a child to begin to master a skill.

- Different types of homework are important for different types of kids. For example, kids who have less knowledge of math concepts learn more when their homework consists of completing small parts of a problem, or doing the problem in a step-by-step fashion while showing their work, while more knowledgeable math students benefit more from working on the entire problem without the need to show their work. Showing your work can be good if you're learning how to do a complex concept (something like long division) and you need to know where in the process you're having difficulty. But if you understand the concept and are getting the correct answer, showing your work can feel tedious and unnecessary. It can sap motivation and a love of math. If your child is struggling with homework, talk to her about why she thinks that's happening and then discuss it with your child's teacher.

- Similarly, students described as "low-level" writers benefit from homework that is more about practicing writing skills, while "high level" writers benefit from "goal-free" homework. Goal-free homework for a child who has good reading skills might be something like "read anything you find pleasurable for 30 minutes a day." If you don't yet know how to read, that "assignment" that's supposed to be building a love of reading won't seem as fun. If you know your child is ready for goal-free homework or needs remediation, talk to your child's teacher about adjusting the homework requirements to support his skill set.

- Programs aimed at encouraging students to read more (reading for 15–30 minutes per day) have not been shown in research to be very effective in boosting reading achievement. Anecdotally, I do not find them all that helpful in instilling a love of reading. They don't take into account that at times we get lost in a book and want to read for hours at a time and at other times we don't feel like reading much at all. To help your child develop a love of reading, be sure that reading is part of your life. Make sure they have access to high-interest books. Reading *good, fun* books that *are about characters like themselves* is the best way to get them interested in reading.

HIGH SCHOOL STUDENTS (GRADES 9 TO 12)

- In contrast to other ages, high school students do appear to benefit from two hours of homework at night, particularly if it is focused on skills that they are learning to master and have a blueprint for how to do, such as completing algebra problems with examples that have been worked out in advance.

- Teens are developmentally ready to spend time on a special talent. Practicing a musical instrument or a sport for one to two hours a day is appropriate for a student at this age. Some of this time will be spent in group practices (orchestra, basketball practice).

- Although programs aimed at encouraging students to read more haven't been shown to be effective, learning new vocabulary words is a good thing to practice. Thus, if you have a high school student who doesn't like to read, no existing program is a sure-fire way to get him to do it, but listening to audiobooks is a good way to learn new vocabulary. Watching and discussing sophisticated movies and TV programs can do the same thing. One of the best predictors of adults who read is having parents who read. Though this is correlational (the two activities are associated, but no one knows if adult reading *causes* kids to read), it's never a bad idea to spend more time reading, at the end of the day, when you're on vacation, or whenever you can. You can't expect your child to pick up a book if you never do so yourself.

THERE'S A RIGHT WAY TO MOTIVATE AND A WRONG WAY: INTRINSIC AND EXTRINSIC MOTIVATION

When parents want their child to practice more, they often pile on the praise or give big incentives. Those types of motivation are called *extrinsic motivators*. They are motivators that come from external factors. In contrast, *intrinsic motivators* are factors that arise from inside of us. Each of these factors has a different effect on a child's behavior and the pursuit of goals.

Extrinsic motivation occurs when we are motivated to do an activity because we want to gain a reward or avoid getting in trouble. It's when we show up for work to a job we don't love because we need a paycheck or when we clean the garage because we are tired of hearing our spouse nagging us about it. Not all extrinsic motivators are bad. We all need a little external push now and then, kids included. Some kids participate in sports to win awards, compete for scholarships, or study to get good grades. Awards and paychecks can help us over the hump when intrinsic motivation is in short supply. The same tasks can be intrinsically motivated—kids participate in sports because they find it fun to do so. You clean the garage because you like to have a clean home. Kids study subjects or compete in challenges because they find a subject fascinating and enjoy solving puzzles.

Studies have shown that while there is a time and place for both intrinsic and extrinsic motivation, offering external rewards for something that's already internally satisfying can reduce intrinsic motivation. Psychology has a term for it—the *overjustification effect*—or the phenomenon that happens when we are offered excessive external rewards for something that is already internally rewarding: *We become less interested.* This concept has been validated in many studies with kids of different ages: *Giving kids a big reward for something sends them the message that it's something that's probably not that fun to do on its own.*

> *Beware of providing external rewards for activities your child already finds internally rewarding—they can turn him off to the activity.*

If you've got a child who doesn't seem to care about anything, you are most likely trying every single external motivator you can think of—money, privileges, social activities, clothes, games, and use of the family car, just to name a few of the most popular ones. You are perhaps completely at a loss for praising your child, and when you do, it might seem insincere or overdone. You increase the extrinsic motivation because you are seeing little to no intrinsic motivation in your child. And then you notice that your attempts at rewarding them to do something, *anything*, don't really work.

Nurturing Intrinsic Motivation

On the other hand, you might not find the idea of intrinsic motivation very compelling. It might seem as if intrinsic motivation works only for kids who actually care about something in the first place. Research, however, doesn't suggest that at all. Or it might be scary to take the plunge from being a parent who relies on external rewards to one who doesn't. One reason is because you are releasing control. And not being in control makes all of us a little nervous, especially if we're talking about a child we fear might crash and burn unless we dangle something tantalizing in front of her. My suggestion is to take this one step at a time. Here are some concrete tips to help you move from being a parent who relies on extrinsic motivation to one who nurtures the intrinsic in your child:

• *Talk to your child about goals.* In Chapter 9 I'll give you more information about why goal setting is an important component for helping kids find a reason to care. Motivated kids have goals. They want good grades, to win a soccer trophy, or to get into medical school. Goals are the reason we care about things, and the best goals are the ones that come from within us. *Talking* to kids about the future is essential to helping them *care* about the future. Ask them what they want. How do they want to spend their time? What do they want to learn this week/month/year in school? What kinds of activities, friends, skills do they want? And DON'T JUDGE. Your child might be interested in things that don't interest you in the least. Encourage him to find his bliss and then find a way to become interested in what he loves.

• *Catch your child doing the right thing.* If you've got a child who couldn't care less, you are likely hyperfocused on what could go wrong. Did your daughter make it to school on time? Did the homework get turned in on time? Did she go to sleep when she said she did, or was she on social media until 2:00 A.M.? If you find yourself always nagging your child because you're worried, try to ignore any behavior that isn't dangerous or won't lead to more problems. In addition, *give your child lots of praise* for doing the right thing. Change the way you communicate with your child to one where you are talking about how they are doing things right and ignoring anything that can be learned through logical consequences. Save your nagging for things that truly need to be said. Ignoring bad behavior is the **best** way to extinguish the behavior, but parents rarely use it.

• *Remind your child that success breeds success.* When you're in the process of learning something, you'll inevitably hit roadblocks and want to quit. Empathize with your children when they feel that way. And then remind them of this truth: *Everything gets better with practice.* If they're having trouble noticing this, give them tangible evidence to the contrary. Help them set smaller goals, ones that are achievable, so they can more easily see their successes.

• *Help your child find things that are intrinsically motivating* and *give them choices.* Kids who don't care typically don't find things like studying interesting for its own sake. They also tend to like things that are outside the box—sports like fencing or karate, chess club, or drama—or they tend not to like what everyone else is doing. Give them a wide berth and (you've heard this before) *don't judge*. If they can't come up with something on their own, give them choices and ideas to get them started. And if they can't make a choice—if there is nothing in the world that interests them—then they may have a bigger problem. Take a look at the information in Chapter 11. Kids might not be intrinsically interested in anything for a number of reasons, such as depression and anxiety. In this case, the first step is figuring out why and finding the appropriate treatment.

• *Don't pile on more pressure.* Once you've listened to your child and he has shown some interest in something, don't make predictions about how great he's going to be at this endeavor. Don't tell him that he's going to be the next Spike Lee just because he's having fun posting short videos he's made on YouTube. Many kids who become apathetic have parents who say things like "He's got a real talent for photography" when all the child has done is open an Instagram account for the family dog. Telling your kid that she is going to "be somebody" is the worst kind of extrinsic motivation—it's unlikely to happen and definitely not going to happen anytime soon. It's the promise of an improbable reward. Heaping praise on children for doing only minimal work or showing just a hint of talent is a near sure-fire way to squelch their interests. Many kids who couldn't care less have parents who have given them loads of (often well-intentioned) lavish praise for the simplest of activities. If this sounds like you, the good news is that it's one of the easiest things to fix.

When to Use Extrinsic Motivation

Remember that extrinsic motivation isn't all bad. It's particularly helpful when we need to finish a task we find unpleasant or when we want to help someone become interested in something new. Here are the best times to use external rewards:

- *When you want to get your child to try something you think they might learn to like.* Maybe you've got an inkling your daughter would enjoy gymnastics, but she's reluctant to try. It's okay to tell her that you'll go out for ice cream if she agrees to try one class. Just remember that if she likes it and starts to go weekly, gymnastics shouldn't be the reason you go out for ice cream after class. Take her out for ice cream because you both like ice cream and you've got time to do it. Most kids are sensitive to their parents' needs, and it's a fine line between having an inkling that you think your child might enjoy something and trying to push your child into doing something you think she should do. Be aware of your own expectations and whether you are providing an external reward or if you're applying pressure.

- *When your child has to do something in a certain time period and he's not interested in doing it.* It could be something like a big project for school or cleaning his room before Grandma visits. Using extrinsic motivation at this time is okay. It's why people feel they're entitled to a beer or soda after they've mowed the lawn and not before.

- *When you want to let your child know she's done something worthy of recognition,* whether it's a good grade on a test or a good game or good effort. Celebrating achievements and giving positive praise can improve intrinsic motivation. These are particularly effective when they are unexpected— like when you decide to order pizza because something good has happened to someone in the family. Just remember to use this sparingly, as you don't want rewards to become something that is expected.

What Kind of Feedback Is Most Effective in Fostering Intrinsic Motivation?

Being a parent means often feeling like you've said the wrong thing. You mean to be helpful, but your child takes the comment as a criticism. You give them rewards, and they don't work (now you know why). You tell them you like what they did, and they tell you they hate it. This is the nature of parenting. Sidestepping the issue ("OK! I just won't say anything!") or being vague ("Well, that's nice") also isn't helpful. Here are a few alternatives that you might find useful:

- Feedback is most effective when you describe how whatever your child has done has met the criteria you expected. For example, you asked your child to pick up his room. Focus on what he did—"You put all of the books on the shelf"—as well as what he could do to improve: "I see you still have a lot of clothes on your bed that need to be hung up." Then provide solutions or support: "Can I help you hang them up?" or "It looks like you're doing great. Let me know if you need more hangers."

- Feedback should be less about you and more about them. Help them reflect on their problem-solving strategy. "Did that way work well for you?"

- Use feedback as a way of helping them reflect on the progress they made and how they feel about it. "Your room looks great. How do you feel?"

Whatever you do, don't give them the "motivational talk." Talking to children about their effort, and the importance of increasing it, is not going to change their behavior. And I mean that with a capital N for *not*. It also doesn't work to ask someone special, like a teacher, to give the talk. In fact, parents ask me all the time to have "the talk" with their child about motivation.

Talking to children about the importance of increasing their effort will not change their behavior.

Xavier's parents were a perfect example. Xavier was a 13-year-old with ADHD who was spending too much time playing video games and too little time completing his homework. I evaluated Xavier and shared the results with his parents. He was bright, but he lacked the executive function skills—the attention, organizational, and self-monitoring skills (see Chapter 1)—that would help him achieve his potential.

"Can you talk to him? He'll listen to you," his parents told me. "Tell him he's got potential. He just has to work harder. He liked you. He'll do it if you tell him he can."

"I really wish it worked that way," I told them. "He's not going to change just because I tell him to do it. But here's what I can do. I can open up a discussion about this. Let's use this as a way to focus on his future performance and to let him know that he has what it takes. I can let him know that we've got some ideas about what might be helpful and that I'm confident that there are things that he'll be able to figure out on his own. I will also ask him to think about what he could do differently and the things that make him happy and feel successful."

Though it wasn't exactly the easy fix his parents wanted, Xavier did come away from the evaluation with a little more insight and some goals. His parents understood that simple motivational lectures weren't ever going to work. When I saw him four years later for a reevaluation before going off to college, they admitted that his success was due to the right supports, the right motivations, and giving him the space to find his passions and to make achievable goals, and not to any motivation speech or big reward.

OVERSCHEDULING

Earlier in the chapter, I told you that there were two major impediments to practicing. One had to do with the type of motivation. The other is overscheduling. Where kids are concerned, schedules are generally very good. From bedtimes for toddlers to homework routines for middle school students, schedules and routines help kids feel in control of their environment. They let them know what is happening now and what to expect tomorrow. Consistent, *appropriate* schedules help kids feel more safe, secure, and comfortable. This allows them to engage more fully in the learning process because they aren't distracted by an uncertain future or unexpected events. Whether it's within the family or school setting, consistency fosters relationships and a sense of belonging and self-confidence.

Notice how I put the word *appropriate* in italics here and in the paragraph above. The kinds of schedules I'm describing are ones that help kids learn routines and develop lifelong habits for things like good sleeping and eating. Schedules, which represent the big picture—the week of activities that happen across the calendar, the routines, the steps needed to complete each part of the schedule—need to be appropriate for a child's age. For a toddler, a schedule is a week filled with bedtimes at 7:30 P.M., a nap in the afternoon, visits to the park in the morning, and regular mealtimes. Routines include reading a story before bed and hanging up coats after returning from the park. For a 12-year-old, a schedule includes school, activities, and time with friends and family. There are a lot of ways to fill in a 12-year-old's schedule, and when the schedule gets packed, routines, like regular bedtimes or mealtimes, are often forgotten.

Lots of kids who are unmotivated at age 14 were overscheduled as early as age six. There have been many books and articles about overscheduling kids (see the list in Chapter 12), and you should take a look at some of them if this is a big issue in your family. I'm mentioning it here because it's a big impediment to practice and to joy. Putting on the persona of not caring about anything becomes children's way out of their overscheduled life—a life of being tired and constantly under pressure. Giving up on everything isn't a good coping skill, but some teens and preteens don't see any other option.

Overscheduling is an impediment to practice—and to joy.

Many overscheduled families are unhappy families, or at least *not*-happy families. There is the constant time in the car. Rushed meals. Lack of sleep. Little sense of mastery despite lots of time in pursuit of it. As overscheduled elementary school students move into high school, they typically move into one of two directions—the adolescent who continues along the path of overscheduling or the child who wants nothing to do with any of it. Embracing overscheduling isn't a good thing for many adolescents, who are at increased risk for anxiety, eating disorders, and depression. For both groups, alcohol and drug use is high. Marijuana use is an epidemic for high school kids, and when they talk to me about it, they all say the same thing—"I need to chill out." In other words, "I've got too much to handle, and this is the best way I can find to relax."

What's it like for them? Instead of giving you an example from a child in my practice, I thought I would share with you an experience I had myself. Maybe there are things in my story that are relatable to you or to your child.

My Middle-Aged Experience as a 12-Year-Old,
or Why Overscheduling Can Lead a Child to Dislike
His Interests and Aptitudes

In the process of writing this book, there was a worldwide pandemic. You might remember this. We all stopped working in offices. Some of you found that you were not cut out for homeschooling. Many confronted medical and health challenges and serious losses. It took us a long time to get back to normal. In the difficult months we all endured, I was quite fortunate. I could do most of my work from home, and I found I had more time on my hands than I did before—or at least I was told I had more time on my hands given that I didn't have to commute or spend moments picking out an outfit every day. I reacted to this event by scheduling myself as if I were a typical U.S. 12-year-old. I added lots of extracurriculars to my calendar. My twice-a-week private Spanish lessons, semester-long course in screenwriting, needlepoint instructions, online workouts, and book clubs, among other things, kept me quite busy. I had something after work almost every day of the week, and that's not counting the weekend conferences on topics ranging from how to write the great American novel to seminars on the best way to DIY your nails (yes, there were seminars on this). I became way overcommitted (and the editor of this book can attest to the fact that it slowed me down in at least one way).

I learned a few things about myself that are easily applied to kids. First, parents hear the suggestion "Don't overdo it. Pick one or two things as extra activities and stick to that." To be honest, few parents heed this advice. But they rarely stop to think what their lives would be like if they had an activity every day after work. I can tell you what it's like. Exhausting. And I didn't have to get into a car and drive 30 minutes to class. There was no time to just "chill," and though a lot of the courses were fun, I always felt behind. There was too much to do, and it was really hard to shift from Spanish class at 5:00 P.M. to a Zoom book club meeting at 7:30, only to need to get to bed early for my 6:30 A.M. fitness class. Unfortunately, this is what we ask kids to do all the time. It really takes the fun out of things that are supposed to be fun.

This experience also taught me something about the Parenting APP. For example, I have no aptitude for learning a foreign language but for a number of different reasons would like to be able to converse in Spanish. Despite not having an aptitude for it, as I practiced Spanish, it became more pleasurable because I started to understand what I was doing. Practicing more subsequently increased my ability/aptitude for learning the language. However, because there were so many other competing activities, it was difficult for me to practice as much as I should have in order to reap the benefits of practice. I'd have some time to practice, and I'd feel more competent, but then remember that I needed to read the book for Tuesday night's book club, and I wouldn't practice Spanish for four days. Much of the pleasure I'd started to feel about Spanish was gone because other things got in the way. Think about this analogy when considering your child's schedule. Sometimes kids simply don't want to practice, but at other times they just are too tired or busy to practice. You might see them start to enjoy an activity that might not have been completely easy for them, and after a brief period of enjoyment they lose interest because they don't have the time for it to become pleasurable. This is one of the main reasons that overscheduling defeats the purpose of helping your child find activities where he can excel.

Oprah has said, "You can have it all. Just not all at once." Although she made the statement about adults, it applies to kids as well. They've got a lifetime to learn all sorts of wonderful things. Give them space and time to enjoy learning or to become competent in one or two things outside the school environment. My brief time as an overscheduled 12-year-old taught me that concentrating on just one or two things at a time would have been much more fun and fruitful.

How Do You Know When Too Much Is Too Much?

The question "How much should my child be doing outside of school?" is one of the most frequent questions I've been asked by parents. They usually ask it because they already know whatever they're doing is already too much. Yet they're afraid to make changes because they don't want their child to be left out of social groups or to miss the chance to become the next Serena Williams. Parents shuttle their kids to tennis lessons, T-ball, ballet, and karate because they want them to be well rounded. To discover their passions. To have a competitive edge. To make friends.

The problem is that overscheduled children are rarely doing any of these things. Yes, they're making friends, but they're often superficial ones that end along with the sports season. Yes, they might be gaining skills, but they come at a cost that might include physical injury due to overuse. They might seem well rounded, but the research shows that most of them will not be karate masters, tennis stars, or concert pianists—and especially not all of these at once. The skills learned from these lessons are things like discipline, a lifelong love of music, and the habit of good physical fitness. Taking classes in something you're interested in learning is something that is good throughout the life span. Keep these things in mind as you're choosing what your child should do.

If you're not sure if your child is overscheduled, here are some of the signs:

- *Loss of interest* in activities they once enjoyed is a frequent sign of an overscheduled child. Did they love Suzuki violin when they were six years old but hate it at age eight because they are in four other activities every week and so they have no time to practice? Do they complain about going to practice?

- *Burnout* is "loss of interest" on a bigger scale—a child who doesn't seem to care about any extracurricular activities. Though it can also be the sign of a bigger problem, most kids who show the initial signs of burnout (seems to hate everything, is grumpy and irritable) are tired and lacking sleep.

- *Changes in sleeping or eating,* especially trouble falling asleep at bedtime, despite not getting enough sleep or overeating as a way to relax.

- *Physical symptoms such as stomachaches, headaches,* or constantly complaining about aches and pains that have no physical cause.

- *Zoning out in front of the TV whenever there is downtime* because they're too tired to do much of anything else.

- *Changes in schoolwork,* such as not finishing homework or slipping grades because there is insufficient time to do homework or because they are too overwhelmed to apply themselves.

- *Your family is constantly stressed and overwhelmed,* and you're worried that you're going to burn out or already have. Are you resentful of the time and money involved in your child's activities? Then it's time to reassess your priorities, as well as your child's.

So what can you do if you've got an overscheduled kid who couldn't care less? And what about the child who doesn't care who now has no activities? The answer is the same—talk to them and listen to what they have to say. If you're in the midst of trying to decide what to keep and what to cut out, your child should be part of the discussion. Pick one or two activities at a time and stick with them. If you're worried that your child will be left out because "everyone" is taking gymnastics, find ways to connect with those kids outside of gymnastics class. You might find that other parents will follow your lead. If you've got a child who was once overscheduled and who now does nothing, start the conversation talking about the past. Typically, these kids are already in middle or high school. Be candid with them. They appreciate when adults own up to mistakes, especially well-intentioned ones. Talk about future goals, about where they'd like to be in five years, and about what makes them happy. As I said earlier, there are great resources on helping families deschedule their lives. Take a look at some of them if you need ideas. They are listed in the back of this book.

If your middle school or high school student has no interest in anything because of being overscheduled for years, own your mistake and start over by talking to your child about what they want.

Final Thoughts on Making Practice Fun

Whether your child needs just a little push to practice or much more structure and encouragement, keep in mind these suggestions:

• *Make it fun.* If they are learning ballet, take them to the ballet. Same goes for live sporting events, concerts, and art galleries. Infusing fun events into their practicing is an enjoyable activity that helps them see the payoff of hard work.

• *Give them the time and space to practice.* Have space in the calendar where they have uninterrupted time to practice without distractions. Sometimes it can be helpful to just leave them alone with their instrument. Many writers swear by the technique of setting aside one hour a day to sit at their computer, ready to write. They consider it part of the "practice" of writing. Sometimes a person might not feel ready to practice, and having time to reflect is enough. Allow that to happen at least once in a while. Make a plan that every day X time is the time for sitting at the piano. If once in a while they sit in silence or improvise silly tunes, it might be a good thing.

• *Practice will make you better,* if not perfect. This is nearly always the case. Doing something more often makes you better at it. Remind children of this fact when they become discouraged. Also remind them of how far they've come. And then find something you love and spend time practicing it yourself. Kids model what they see in their lives.

The Parenting APP

On the next page is what the completed Parenting APP looks like. If you haven't spent time filling in these sections, spend some time now thinking about it. Writing down your child's attributes and behaviors can make things seems more tangible and manageable. Pay particular attention to where these areas intersect.

Complete Venn Diagram for the Parenting APP

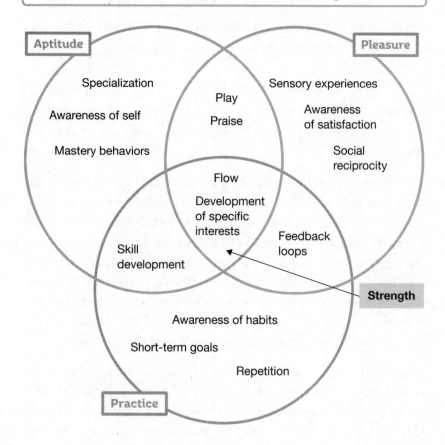

THINK, TALK, DO

 What to Think About

- What activities does your child return to without adult prompting?
- What kind of feedback does your child typically get from you and the other adults around her?
- When your child needs to practice or do homework, what kind of structure is in play to support him? Is it too much or too little?

- What kinds of rewards do you typically give? How comfortable are you with letting your child find an intrinsic reward? What kinds of extrinsic rewards are you giving? Are they appropriate?

- Is your child overscheduled? If so, what could be changed?

What to Talk About

- Ask your child:
  - How do you like spending your time? Is there anything you could do over and over and not get bored?
  - What do you wish you had the skills to do? What kind of activities do you wish you could do?
  - What do you want to learn this week/month/year in school?
  - What kinds of assignments do you enjoy completing? What assignments do you absolutely hate doing?

- Talk to your child about the kinds of tasks that need a "push" (an external reward) and figure out what that task would look like when finished, along with an appropriate reward.

- Make a list of the activities your child does in a typical week and talk about each one. Ask questions such as:
  - What do you enjoy about this activity?
  - What do you wish you could change about this activity?
  - What's missing from this list? Are there other things you'd like to be doing?
  - What should we eliminate?

What to Do

- Practice giving feedback that fosters intrinsic motivation.

- If your family is overscheduled, make changes to your life so that you're less stressed.

- Remind your child about the "end goals" of practice.

- When your child finds something intrinsically motivating, avoid piling on the praise or pressure.

- Spend time reading (the whole family, not just your child) or listening to audiobooks. Poor reading and vocabulary skills can limit a child's choices in finding pleasurable activities they want to practice.

PART II

Knowing Your Child— and Yourself

Why Understanding Your Child's Unique Qualities Is Important

Part I of this book explored the Parenting APP—*aptitude, pleasure, and practice*—and these concepts are a great place to begin to understand why lots of kids couldn't care less. Interspersed in that discussion were some ideas about what you can do. I'll also provide you with specific techniques that have been shown to motivate difficult-to-motivate kids in Part III of this book. But between the APP and Part III are an individual child, with a specific personality, your own personality, and your expectations. We'll explore these factors in this and the next two chapters. I want to be clear that none of this is simple. A specific personality type or a specific event will not typically in and of itself cause a child to lose motivation. But understanding the factors that might cause a child to care or not care can not only help you understand potential causes of the problem but also provide clarity about the solution.

Some of these factors can be seen at a child's birth, while others develop over time. A child's personality influences how we view our kids. Sometimes our kids "click" with our personality, and at other times they don't. More often than not, kids who don't seem to care about anything fall into the second group—the kids who don't click with their mom or dad or the rest of the family. That's not always the case, however. Sometimes the easy baby becomes the difficult preteen, and parents aren't prepared for the adjustment. Regardless, personality counts—both yours and your child's.

Think of these next three chapters as a bridge between the APP and the solutions. In this chapter, we'll explore the ways that temperament and personality play a role in motivation and parenting styles. In the next chapter, I will discuss how parental and societal expectations cause lots of kids to give up. In Chapter 8, we'll explore how parenting styles can play a role in why a child might lose motivation—and how knowledge of one's parenting styles can be used to develop solutions.

How Temperament Influences Motivation

There is wide variability in how children respond to different situations. Watch any preschool classroom on the very first day of school and you'll find that some kids will eagerly rush through the classroom door and others will wait to watch what happens to those who went in first. Still others will cling to an adult and refuse to participate at all. How young children react to the world around them is a complex interplay of biology, environment, and learning. The biological aspect of this is often referred to as *temperament*. In the 1960s child psychiatrists Alexander Thomas and Stella Chess were two of the first researchers to study the idea of temperament.

The baby you might describe as having a certain temperament can become a child you would describe quite differently thanks to the child's experiences over the years.

perament. Their research indicated there are three categories of temperament in young children: *easy, difficult,* and *slow to warm up.* Since then, other researchers have expanded the definition of temperament to include things like emotional and attentional reactivity, or how intensely a child reacts to her environment. While infant temperament is generally thought to be genetically based and fairly stable, how children react and behave as they continue to develop is shaped by environmental experiences. So, temperament is less stable the older we get.

Why is temperament important to consider when you have a child who couldn't care less? Because some of the issues you're struggling with

Temperament is the general behavioral style that determines how we react to situations and express and regulate our emotions. Experts don't all agree on how these characteristics might predict the person we eventually become, but when we are talking about temperament and childhood behaviors, we are referring to things like activity level, distractibility, adaptability, sensitivity, and quality of mood.

may have started long before you ever considered how homework completion would affect your family. Because taking your child's temperament into account will help you interact better with him. For example, if you have a child who is temperamentally not easily able to adapt to new things in the environment, it's likely he'll be more distressed by change, especially sudden change. A more consistent schedule or preparing him for the changes you know about in advance might be good ways to make him less negative. Similarly, if you know that you have a child who is temperamentally irritable, knowing (and remembering) this fact can make you more likely to support her and control her environment in ways that won't escalate her behavior.

I met Andy and his parents for the first time when he was six. Andy was his parents' second child. His older sister, Amy, was described as an "easy" baby who was predictable and calm. "We could take her anywhere!" Andy's mom told me. "Then we got Andy, and we haven't been anywhere since. We love him, but our family has never been the same. It's difficult for us to travel, because he's a picky eater and he doesn't sit still even when it's food that he likes."

Andy's dad added, "He's not just picky about food; he's picky about everything. His socks have to be just right. The tags have to be cut off his shirts, and it's got to be done perfectly. And these are all distractions for him. When it's time for him to do his homework, he can spend 30 minutes getting the seam of his sock perfectly in line with his toes. I leave him alone, thinking he's working on writing sentences for his spelling words, and all he's done is play with his socks. I can't get him to care about anything that's important."

I asked them to tell me a little bit more about what Andy was like as a baby. "In a word, difficult," his mom said. "I could never get him on a schedule. The slightest noise could wake him up, but then other times it seemed he could sleep all day if I'd let him. Anything could set him off—the wrong kind of chicken nuggets or telling him it was time to leave the playground— he'd throw a fit."

Andy sounded like a child with a challenging temperament. As his parents explained more to me, it became clear that his tendency to have trouble adjusting to a different brand of chicken nuggets showed up in all sorts of problems once school started—trouble adjusting to new teachers, new students, and new assignments. Andy's way of coping was to tune out. A difficult, hypersensitive child was becoming a child who seemed to not care about anything, and his parents were worried.

Temperament is typically evidenced early in development. Kids who are at the extremes of these traits are given labels such as "shy," "outgoing," or "difficult" before they reach the age of one or two years. Labels like these can become self-fulfilling prophecies. If you—or relatives, friends, and teachers—use them, come up with other ways of describing your child. I've heard many parents describe their children as "tough" or "difficult" or "a handful" or "troubled." Terms like these are useful for me to get an understanding of family dynamics and history. They are less useful for people like teachers, who will be working intensely with a child over a long period of time, as they can lead to negative expectations. These sorts of labels may contribute to behavioral and emotional difficulties in later years, especially difficulties associated with being unmotivated. Andy's parents started to use the word *discerning* instead of *picky* to define Andy's tendency to like things "just so." As he matured, he started to embrace this quality. It turned out he did like a lot of foods, but he needed time to look at and smell them—to check them out—before he felt like tasting them. Armed with the idea that he wasn't *picky* but was *sensitive* and *discerning*, what was once a negative became a more of a positive. This alone did not turn Andy from a child who didn't care to one who did, but it was an important piece of the puzzle. I've met a lot of kids in their late teens who were still picky eaters—or bad sleepers—or labeled *shy, slow, difficult*. It's hard to care about almost anything

Negative labels for aspects of temperament can become self-fulfilling prophecies.

when you think of yourself as difficult. None of the ideas in this book will work well if your child is still living with labels that make him feel bad about himself.

Whether you are the parent of a three-year-old or a 17-year-old, it's not too late to change the way you describe your child's temperament. It's not that your description was wrong. It's just that the labels themselves take on a life of their own. You probably have 50 things you could say to describe your child right off the top of your head, but the ones that stick around (sometimes far into adulthood) are the negative ones. The chart on page 122 gives you alternatives for some of the more common words we use to describe kids' temperaments. It is far from an exhaustive list, but it can help you think about the other side of any label.

Even the most negative labels have upsides. It's okay if your child knows he's often irritable; it's just better to say to him, "Some kids feel things more deeply and quicker than others, and those kids are more prone to feeling irritable more often," rather than "You're always so irritable, and you make the rest of the family walk on eggshells." It's okay for kids to know that other people tend to walk on eggshells around them, if that indeed is true, but it needs to be discussed in the context of something like, "We love you so much that we would do anything to not see you unhappy. It makes us feel anxious, almost to the point where we are afraid to do anything. What can we do to make us both feel less anxious and irritable?"

There are positive aspects to each type of temperament. The key to a happy adulthood is to find situations and activities that play to our strengths. Highly emotional, reactive kids sometimes find a niche in the arts or theater. Is your child a drama queen? Think about whether a theater class might be a good niche. Is your child shy and introverted? Think about whether she has the calm,

Reframing temperament labels positively can help children find situations and activities that play to their strengths, thus motivating them and leading to a happy adulthood.

REFRAMING YOUR LANGUAGE

Negative	Positive
Difficult	Strong-willed
Shy	Self-reflective
Impulsive	Curious
Introverted	Calm and introspective
Picky	Discerning
Bossy	Determined
Tough	Resolute
Distractible	Perceptive
Unfocused	Exploring
Obsessive	Passionate
Unsociable	Self-reliant
Slow	Easy-going
Indifferent	Consistent
Annoying	Persistent

self-regulated temperament that might enjoy taking care of the neighbors' animals, younger children, or doing something more reflective like joining a parent–child book club.

The Five-Factor Theory of Personality

One of the most widely used and best-studied models of personality is the five-factor theory of personality. These five broad personality traits are *extraversion* (sometimes spelled extroversion), *agreeableness, openness, conscientiousness,* and *neuroticism.* Each of these personality factors represents a range between two opposite extremes. For example, extraversion is really a continuum between extraversion and introversion. Most of us lie somewhere in between these two poles. These five categories are often described in the following ways.

OPENNESS

Openness is a trait for which the opposite pole is *closed to experience*. It features characteristics such as imagination and curiosity. People who are high in this trait tend to be more adventurous and sometimes even more unconventional. People low in this trait tend to be more traditional and to dislike change. They might resist trying out new ideas. A child who is too far at either extreme might have difficulties and also opportunities. Too much openness to experience makes you eager to climb to the highest spot on the jungle gym at age two, which is great for developing motor skills but not so great when the exploration leads to a broken arm. Too little openness makes it difficult to get excited about going to a friend's birthday party, even when it's something you know you'd enjoy.

In the first example of the jungle gym, a child might decide that the experience was too traumatic, resulting in their no longer wanting to go to the park. Or the parent might decide that climbing is too dangerous. In either case, the child is not doing what he naturally enjoyed doing. Unless that's replaced with something else that's equally enjoyable, that child might become one who spends more time in front of a screen than in the park. In the second example of the child who has trouble with birthday parties, the effect can be a child who stops getting invited to parties, whose world shrinks to just a few kids or even one or none. None of these things are typically sudden game changers, but some parents can point back to a time or situation that was difficult, didn't get any better, and slowly changed the child's world in ways that led them to not care much about anything. One of the most common experiences is of the naturally gifted athletic child who suffers a setback from an injury, losing not only the sport they loved but also the peer group who goes on to play without them. This can happen even quite early in development, though it's more common in middle and high school.

CONSCIENTIOUSNESS

People high in the trait of *conscientiousness* tend to be organized and to like to plan ahead. They love deadlines and assignments. This is a trait that increases over the life span. Young children aren't typically very high in this trait, but you can see it developing in them when you notice them trying to control their impulses. Adolescents who are high in conscientiousness tend to be self-disciplined and to strive for achievement. On the other end of the spectrum is a *lack of direction*. People with low conscientiousness tend to be less disciplined. They dislike schedules and structure and don't mind a mess. Being at either end of these traits can be too much of a good thing (a student who spends too much time preparing for a test) or too little (a child who procrastinates about studying for a test). Either one of these can interfere with motivation. Studying too much for a test isn't fun, which can make the subject seem less fun too, interfering with the intrinsic motivation of a love of learning the subject. If overstudying is paired with subsequent poor test performance, it can make a student feel like "what's the use?" Not studying for a test can also lead to poor grades—and poor grades are not just an outcome but also a cause of poor motivation. It's hard to find motivation for something that you've failed.

EXTRAVERSION

Extraversion is the trait that you're probably already somewhat familiar with, as its polar opposite is introversion. People high in extraversion tend to be sociable, talkative, and emotionally expressive, but more importantly, they gain energy in social situations. *Introverts* tend to be more reserved, but more importantly, they are depleted by social situations. You can be an outgoing introvert, but you'll need to have time to charge your batteries. If you've got a 10-year-old who is always the life of the party but then just wants to stay in his room and chill for a weekend after a week of holiday parties, you might have a sociable introvert. Extraverts love to start conversations and to meet new people, and they find it easy to make new friends. They are invigorated when around other people. Introverts prefer solitude, hate small talk, and need time alone to re-charge after having lots of social contact. The extraverted child might be exposed to a lot of new experiences because she likes learning things with others, but she might also be more prone to flit from activity to activity because she likes the social interactions that come from joining a team or a class. The introverted child might be good at persisting in one interest while spending a lot of time alone, free to decide where to put his energies. On the other hand, the introverted child might have a tougher time if he's been living for an activity like chess club and there aren't enough kids to continue it.

AGREEABLENESS

The trait of *agreeableness* includes abilities such as trust, kindness, compliance, and altruism. People high in agreeableness tend to be more cooperative, while those low in this trait (with the other end of the spectrum considered a lack of agreeableness or even *antagonism*) tend to be more competitive and sometimes even controlling. Children who are high in agreeableness tend to show a lot of interest in other people and enjoy helping and contributing to the happiness of others. Kids who are low in this trait can be difficult and even manipulative in getting what they want. This trait doesn't start to become stable until adolescence, and it increases throughout adulthood. Two-year-olds tend to be lopsided in this trait—it's what makes them the terrible twos—but they grow out of it, becoming more agreeable as they mature, or at least that is the goal of mature behavior. But you don't have to have this trait in spades to be a successful adult. Competitiveness and being less agreeable have their place in society. It's more about knowing where you fall on this trait. If a child seems to be low in this trait, you might need to point out ways to be empathic and helpful to others, as well as how to be less demanding. Kids who are low in agreeableness might lose motivation when they're in situations where they feel they can't win or where their tendency to be less agreeable makes them not as well liked by their peers.

NEUROTICISM

Finally, *neuroticism* is best thought of as, well, being a bit neurotic. This can include having a tendency toward anxiety, irritability, moodiness, and sadness. People who are high in neuroticism tend to be more self-consciousness and less self-confident. The opposite is *emotional stability*, or a person who deals well with stress, doesn't worry about things that they don't need to worry about, and is generally more relaxed. People who are high in neuroticism tend to have difficulty bouncing back after stressful events and tend to spend time needlessly worrying. Kids high in neuroticism might be prone to losing motivation because they are worried about their performance or be too self-conscious to participate in activities, even ones they enjoy doing.

Virtually all temperament traits have an upside and a downside—to motivate your child, find the upside.

PERSONALITY AS A MOVING TARGET

Although we can get a fairly good sense of where we stand on these personality traits as adults, in kids these traits are evolving. Extraversion increases over the first year (a baby becomes a more outgoing toddler) and then decreases from early to middle childhood. Extraversion generally decreases over the course of adulthood. Babies start out with a fair amount of negative emotionality (neuroticism). Those tendencies decrease beginning in late adolescence or early adulthood. Agreeableness is one trait that tends to be somewhat stable until adolescence but increases across adulthood. Conscientiousness is something that increases in childhood, though the findings are mixed for conscientiousness in adolescence. Openness to experience tends to increase in some people through early adulthood and then decrease in later life.

These findings show that although we have tendencies, they are influenced by our age and the world in which we live. And the influence doesn't work in just one direction. Temperament characteristics influence the environment, with certain characteristics leading some children to seek out certain environments (taking a harder course load) and to alter or modify those environments (getting more or less attention from a teacher, which causes a student to be more or less agreeable or conscientious).

Understanding Your Child's Temperament and Your Own

So, what does all of this mean for you and your child? It might be good to spend some time thinking about where your child falls in these traits now and where *you* fall. Are you an introverted parent who is constantly exhausted by an extraverted child who needs your attention? Are you an adult who is highly open to new experiences but has a child who dislikes change? Perhaps both you and your child are very conscientious, and it makes for a lot of anxiety in the household. Or is one of you highly neurotic and stressed and the other never gets rattled, even when it's appropriate to be anxious? Knowing how your child's personality fits with yours and the rest of the family's can help you not only understand some aspects of why your child couldn't care less but also find the best way to interact positively with your child to guide her toward being more motivated.

Fill out the grid on "What Is Your Temperament? What Is Your Child's Temperament?" (page 128). (You can also download and print this form from *www.guilford.com/braaten4-forms*.) Do you match? Where do you differ? For more information, take one of the tests listed in the "What to Do" section at the end of this chapter. Do one for yourself and imagine what your child would say. If you have a child who is old enough to take the test themselves, do it together and see where you differ. It's a great way to open up a dialogue about accepting who you are and accepting the differences in others.

Personality and temperament are important traits in understanding you and your child, but they're only a start. Temperaments are born and nurtured in environments. I don't need to tell you that the environments kids are living in today bear little resemblance to the environment in which you were raised. On top of this are the lasting effects of being a child during a long worldwide pandemic. In the next chapter, I'll cover some of the more difficult 21st-century challenges of child-rearing—school stress and what is considered the pot at the end of the rainbow, admission to a great college—as well as the most common parenting styles that (even when well-intentioned) can lead kids to not caring. But before we get there, here are

What Is Your Temperament? What Is Your Child's Temperament?

		I am:	My child is:
Openness	More curious/imaginative		
	Less curious/imaginative		
	More practical		
	Less practical		
Conscientiousness/ effortful control	Highly attentive		
	Less attentive		
	Highly controlled		
	Less controlled		
Extraversion/ surgency	Highly active		
	Less active		
	Very shy		
	Less shy		
	Highly impulsive		
	Less impulsive		
Neuroticism/ negative affectivity	More easily frustrated		
	Less easily frustrated		
	Hard to soothe when upset		
	Easier to soothe when upset		
	Often fearful or anxious		
	Less often fearful or anxious		
Agreeableness	More compassionate/helpful		
	Less compassionate/helpful		
	More trusting/less suspicious		
	Less trusting/more suspicious		

some ways to think about and explore the ideas of temperament and personality.

THINK, TALK, DO

What to Think About

- How is your temperament similar to your child's? How is it different?
- What kind of temperament did your child have as a baby? How has that changed (or not) over time?
- How do you typically react to stressful situations with your child? Are you slow to anger? Or too quick? How do your reactions change the outcome of their behaviors?
- What activities are best suited to your child's temperament? How many of those activities are currently in his schedule?
- What activities are *not* well-suited to your child's temperament? If those activities are necessary (group work for an introverted child), how can you best support them?
- What language do you use to describe your child? How can you reframe the negative language?

What to Talk About

- Ask your child:
  - How would you describe our family? How is that description similar or different from yourself?
  - What makes your personality special?
  - What are five words you'd use to describe yourself?
- Do one of the tests listed below with your child and talk about the results. Fill in the grid listed earlier in this chapter and discuss how you differ and are the same.

What to Do

- Fill out the grid "What Is Your Temperament? What Is Your Child's Temperament?" on page 128.

- Take some tests that measure the five personality factors mentioned in the chapter. Some good (and free!) links include:

  - *https://openpsychometrics.org/tests/IPIP-BFFM*
  - *www.psychologistworld.com/influence-personality/five-factor-test*
  - *https://my-personality-test.com/big-5*

SEVEN

How Your Expectations Can Get in the Way

When I was pregnant with my first child, I had a conversation over coffee with a group of other first-time expectant mothers. We were discussing how we would be happy with *anything* our child would be. As we got to know each other better, many of us shared that we had been raised to think we either weren't qualified to do the things we wanted to do or that we *shouldn't* do the things we wanted to do. We were planning to raise our children *very* differently. As we shared our stories of things we'd been told, they went something like this: "Who majors in art? You'll never be able to support yourself as an artist!" Or "Math isn't your thing. You will never make it in medical school." Or "If you want me to help you with graduate school, I'm not paying for a PhD in English. If you want to go to law school, that's fine, but I'm not signing loans for you to read books for four years." And then there were others who were told, "Sorry, we don't have the money for college. You'll have to let that dream go for now." Or "I don't think you have a head for school. Working in your dad's store is a better plan."

Expectations—Great and Not So Great

Yes, as we sat there talking about the wonderful opportunities that awaited our unborn children, we asked each other, "Can you imagine anything your child would want to do that you wouldn't support?" As I shook my head, a thought popped into my mind: "an accountant." I have no idea why. I love my accountant. I would be lost without him. It looks like a fabulous career path, except for the month of March and half of April. But at that moment, I realized I had a dream that my child would be more than a person who sits in an office managing money. I had a dream she would be a game-changer, an artist, perhaps the second female president of the United States (assuming there was already a first). A female conductor of the Boston Symphony! A novelist. A CEO.

Many of us have these dreams. There's nothing wrong with them—in fact, they are a wonderful part of being a parent—but they can cloud our judgment when reality sets in. They can put a lot of unneeded pressure on kids. Learning to parent the child we have—not the child we dreamed about—is one of our greatest challenges as parents. For some of us, it can be very disappointing to find out that our kids will be like nearly every other child who grows into adulthood—*normal*.

What sort of expectations do you have for your child? These expectations might have taken root before your child was even conceived. Many of us became parents because we had dreams of babies and baseball practices and loving someone in new and wonderful ways. How have your expectations changed since you first dreamed of having a baby? What do you expect your child will be doing next year? In five years? In ten years? Do you see them as an adult?

These aren't just hypothetical questions. They are important because clashes between what you hope your child will be and what your child is capable of being—or wants to be—often underlie the problematic behaviors of kids who couldn't care less. And those aren't the only questions worth asking. Examine your own life. What are the experiences you had in your childhood that you hope your child will have? What experiences do you hope your child will avoid having?

I posed some of these questions to Ryan, dad of 14-year-old Megan. Ryan had been a very good hockey player in high school. In fact, he almost went pro, and he did it without much support from his family. His dad was a lawyer who also happened to be an alcoholic. When he wasn't working, he was drinking, and if he had time for sports, it was golf, not a sport like hockey. As a boy, Ryan wished he'd had the kind of dad who coached his hockey team—or at the very least a dad who consistently came to his games. When Megan was born, Ryan had her on the ice soon after she was able to walk. He coached every one of her hockey teams and was happy that Megan showed some potential. She wasn't a superstar on the ice, but she was good. "With practice—lots of practice—she could have been great," he told me.

Ryan shared with me that when Megan was in fourth grade she had a minor concussion when she slipped on the ice and hit the back of her head. She didn't lose consciousness, but she felt a little dizzy for a day or two and was told not to play hockey for a few weeks. A couple months later she accidentally hit her head on a diving board. She didn't tell anyone about it right away but then started complaining about difficulty concentrating. She attributed it to a pickup game of touch football when she was visiting her cousins a few weeks before. She underwent a number of evaluations, and her neurologist suggested she take a break from sports for a season. When she went back to hockey in sixth grade, she continued to complain about problems related to the previous concussions. She was an honorary member of the hockey team, but she didn't practice with them. She started to complain that the girls on the hockey team were mean to her. When one of the girls said in an offhand comment, "If I wasn't playing, I'd be afraid I'd gain weight like you did," Megan became depressed. She refused to go to school, complaining about migraine headaches that made it impossible for her to concentrate.

When Megan's parents came to me, they were devastated. Her dad thought she'd be a Division 1 athlete in college. Now he was afraid she wasn't going to finish eighth grade, let alone high school. Megan arrived in my office as a wonderful, intelligent adolescent who spent much of her free time writing short stories and poetry. She confessed to me that it was a relief not to play hockey anymore, but underneath her happy exterior was a young girl who was extremely anxious and unhappy. Before she was forced to quit hockey, almost all her free time revolved around the sport. Now all she had was free time, and it was making her depressed. I worked with Megan on her journey into high school. It was a complicated one that included medication, cognitive-behavioral therapy that helped her manage physical and emotional symptoms of anxiety, and a school placement that better suited her.

Most of the work centered around Megan, but some of the change needed to happen with her parents. They were worried they were, in their words, "bad parents." I assured them they were not. They had raised her the best way they knew how. It might have worked perfectly if Megan hadn't had the back luck of having multiple concussions. This "bad luck" happened at a crucial time in her development and required the entire family to regroup in a way they were not prepared to do. While some families with kids who couldn't care less tell me their children have been this way their entire lives, others find themselves in a situation such as this—needing to reassess their expectations. In every case, the challenge for parents is in knowing how to *raise the child you have*, not the child you wish you'd had or the child you had before a life-changing event occurred.

What Are Your Expectations for *Your* Child?

Parental expectations refer to how far you *believe* or *expect* your child *will* go. You can have expectations for education, sports, careers, their future, and all sorts of other things that you deem important. Expectations differ from *aspirations*, which are how far you *want* your child to go. While we may use these terms interchangeably every day, they're not quite the same. Or at least they shouldn't be. Expectations, when they are appropriate for the child, should be based on a realistic assessment of a child's ability and opportunities (remember what you learned about aptitude and pleasure in Chapters 3 and 4). In a perfect world, expectations change as your knowledge of your child's strengths and weaknesses becomes better informed. Aspirations tend to remain stable, despite the evidence to the contrary. That means that even though your child might display

> *Aspirations are about what we hope our children will do or become; expectations are what we believe they can and will do or become.*

no talent or interest in playing the piano, you still might wish or aspire for them to play.

For example, Claudia's parents were both doctors, and their aspirations were that Claudia would become a doctor too or, at the very least, get an advanced degree in some scientific field. Their expectations were the same. They wanted Claudia to be an adult with an MD or a PhD behind her name, and they expected her to perform at a high level in math and science classes. When Claudia was diagnosed with a significant math disability in sixth grade that could make it particularly challenging for her to do medical school—or even high school algebra—with ease, they had trouble changing their aspirations as well as their expectations. Claudia's difficulty with math made her feel like she was a failure in her parents' eyes. Her parents thought that with the right tutoring and support, she would enjoy math more and she would master any challenges. As Claudia progressed into high school, the pressure they'd put on her to excel in a subject that was difficult for her led her to cope in the best way she could—by rejecting school altogether and seeming as if she didn't care about anything.

Imagine this scene a little differently. Imagine that when Claudia was evaluated in sixth grade, her parents used the information from the evaluation to revise their expectations. Imagine they focused their energy on getting Claudia the right support and communicating with her about what she needed to be successful. Along with that, instead of expecting Claudia to perform at the level they deemed important for success, they empathized with her and changed their expectations based on her ability and interests. This does not mean that Claudia is off the hook for math. To the contrary. Having realistic expectations would more likely increase the probability that Claudia might find math worthy of studying, perhaps even as a med student one day. It's not completely unusual for kids with dyslexia to become writers and editors and kids with math disabilities to become scientists. Many of us are drawn to the challenge of overcoming our weaknesses. The difference is that we were allowed to try and fail. We

Even if our aspirations for our kids stay the same, we have to be ready to change our expectations to match reality.

were given the correct support when we failed (or at least we knew where we could go for support). The bar wasn't too high or too low but was achievable.

HOW UNREALISTIC EXPECTATIONS CAN LEAD TO LOW MOTIVATION

When I talk to parents about their expectations for their children, many have shared with me that they have high expectations because they feel that if they don't, their child won't be successful. Parents hear this from teachers, other parents, and the media. Trends in the United States over the last 20 years show that parents' expectations are the highest they've ever been. My own experiences working with schools in India, Singapore, the Middle East, and Europe lead me to believe that these trends are shared with upwardly mobile parents from many places around the world. What would some of the statistics indicate? In multiple studies, very high numbers of parents (over 90% in some studies) expected their children to attain education beyond high school. Over half of all parents expect their child to obtain a bachelor's degree or higher. Nearly all parents believe their child will have more opportunities to thrive and succeed than they did.

Are these high expectations good or bad? It depends. High academic expectations in the *adolescents themselves* are associated with better mental health, but that's only an association. In other words, when kids say "I want to go to Harvard—or be captain of the track team," they are more likely to have good mental health than are kids who don't care about being captain of the track team. It might be that good mental health leads to higher aspirations, not the other way around. High *parental* aspirations are associated with higher academic achievement in kids, but the relationship between those parental aspirations and mental health isn't so clear. For example, parents who say "my child will be a doctor" tend to have kids who do go further in their education, but they might not be so happy while they're getting there. Some studies have indicated that high parental expectations are associated with kids who are stressed about meeting those expectations. Those kids are at increased risk of anxiety and depression. On the other hand, *low* expectations aren't the answer. Saying "you'll never amount to anything" is never helpful. In fact, when parents and kids have low expectations, the child is more likely to have problems with aggression, delinquency, and oppositionality. So, expectations that are too high or too low can be associated with a child who couldn't care less at some point in time.

Your child can end up unmotivated when your expectations are too high or too low.

Other studies show the association between expectations and achievement are more nuanced. It might not be the expectations but the parental criticism that often accompanies expectations that leads to negative mental health outcomes in students. For example, Shayla's parents had high hopes that she would go into law or medicine like most of the rest of her family, but the way they attempted to motivate her was to say things like "If you don't get better grades, you'll never get into a good college and law school will be out of the question." The hopes they had might have been good, but their criticisms led to her losing motivation.

HOW YOUR RELATIONSHIP WITH YOUR CHILD AFFECTS MOTIVATION

The quality of the parent–child relationship is also important to consider. When relationships are strained, higher expectations can have a much more negative impact than when there is a close parent–child bond. Shayla had never had what she felt was a close relationship with her parents. She had been a difficult baby, while her older brother, Ted, was noted to be the "easy one." Ted was particularly close to his father, so his father's criticisms didn't affect Ted's feelings too much. "My dad is just like that," he'd say to anyone who asked about the pressure his parents put on him. Shayla, because she lacked that close connection, felt quite differently about her dad and herself as well.

Most importantly, when high expectations are accompanied by parents who are responsive to what a child needs, the child is more likely to have better mental health. Better communication and a close relationship can alleviate some of the stress of high parental aspirations, as it did for Ted.

Problems most frequently occur when there are differences in what the child and the parent want. It's particularly difficult on kids when parents have higher aspirations than their kids do—and when those aspirations are unrealistic. It can lead to children who couldn't care less.

EXPECTATIONS THAT MATCH THE CHILD YOU HAVE

By now, you are probably thinking "So what is a parent to do?" My advice is to try to be more attuned to your child's aspirations and more aware of your own expectations. Be open to revising your aspirations and expectations as you learn more about your child's interests and abilities. Think about forming expectations that will put your child in that sweet spot of flow we talked about in Chapter 4—where high ability meets just the right amount of challenge. That's where kids get motivated and expectations are more likely to be met. Here are some ways to get there:

• *Spend time talking to your child about your expectations and theirs.* I find that so often these important topics are communicated in anger and frustration. "You'll never go to college with grades like this!" or "I can't imagine you ever living independently!" are sometimes the only kinds of conversations parents have with their kids about college until junior year of high school. If you're screaming these sorts of things to your child, take a step back and start a discussion about your expectations and his. Think about the aptitudes and strengths that you identified in Chapter 3. And don't wait until you're at the point of yelling at your child. Have discussions early—definitely by middle school. Talk about your hopes for their future and your expectations about college and adulthood. If you have the kind of child who shows no interest in going to college, make another plan. Moreover, support your child's self-directed efforts to succeed.

• *Trust the feedback from teachers,* and if you don't trust the teacher, find someone with knowledge about your child you can trust. What do I mean by trusting the feedback? If teachers say things like "I don't see how he'll be ready for kindergarten . . . or college," don't immediately think they are wrong. If your child is getting D's, but you don't trust the teacher's assessment, you won't be dissuaded from thinking your child is on the way to Harvard (or kindergarten). This does not mean that every teacher is correct. And sometimes teachers can single out students they don't like and do everything they can to undermine your child's motivation. I'm not talking about those teachers (who it goes without saying should not be in the profession in the first place). I'm talking about using the valid feedback from trusted professionals to develop appropriate expectations. Before the 2020 pandemic, it was fairly common for parents to challenge my testing results or the informal assessment of teachers. Statements like "He's not *that* inattentive" or "I don't see him as hyperactive; he's just a boy" were made as facts by parents with high expectations. With the necessity for remote learning during COVID-19, it didn't take long for parents to come back to me and say "I had no idea how hard it was for my child to pay attention" or "He's not keeping up with the rest of the class. I can see what they're doing, and he's really far behind." As horrible as the pandemic was, it provided an opportunity for parents to gain insight into their children's abilities, allowing them to set more realistic expectations along with providing more appropriate support.

• *Know the difference between talent and hard work* and understand that you can influence one and not the other. I've seen a lot of really smart, talented kids become kids who couldn't care less because they were raised in an environment (school and/or home) that believed that their academic, artistic, or athletic talents were all that mattered. Make sure you have expectations for *how* they are going to reach the expectations you've set. The *how* is usually more about the work than the talent. Think about the answer to the question posed in Chapter 5: *What does your child persist at?* If he's not persisting at things that he seems to love and has an aptitude for, find ways to support the hard work that is always part of success.

• *Have a realistic understanding of your child's capabilities.* As I said above, remote learning had a big effect on parents' understanding of their child's abilities. Some parents expressed concern that their child wasn't being challenged, and others were amazed that their child was able to be successful in any environment. Many of these parents over- or underestimated what their child could do. If your child has learning challenges, get more information on what those are. Making the mistake of thinking your child is more or less capable than she really is underlies many of the problems with expectations.

Goodness of Fit

Goodness of fit is the match between a child's temperament/personality and the environment. If you've got more than one child, you might have found that one child's temperament seemed to fit naturally into your family while another child's did not. It's not about one child being *difficult*. Any trait in and of itself isn't a problem. Instead, it's the interaction that determines whether the child's behavior is problematic or not.

There are two types of goodness of fit—how the trait acts with the *environment* and how the trait interacts with the *people in the environment*. Research has shown that a goodness of fit between a child's temperament and parenting style is important for healthy social and emotional development. A good fit means that the parents match their demands or expectations with their child's temperament. It's a tough thing to do because creating a good fit means you need to meet not only the needs of that particular child but also the needs of everyone else in the family (including your own). It's worth the effort, though, as when parents' expectations and demands aren't a good fit for the child, it can lead to stress in the parent–child relationship and children who develop behavior problems. What did you learn in Chapter 6 about your child's personality and how it fit with your own personality? Is there a goodness of fit, or are your temperaments so different that it's going to take some work for you to be able to meet your child's needs?

Knowing your child's temperament and personality is a key ingredient in fostering any parent–child relationship, but it

> Your child will be more likely to get motivated when there is goodness of fit between the child and the environment, between the child and you, between your expectations and the child you have.

is particularly essential when you have a child who doesn't care. Unfortunately, when a child has reached the point of not caring, the ability to have a realistic (particularly positive) view of a child's temperament is clouded by frustration and anger. "What does it matter what he was like as a baby? So what if he was shy and slow to warm up?" parents will ask me. "I just want him to find something that interests him. I want him to be excited about going to social events." Understanding goodness of fit isn't going to be a magic bullet that solves all your problems, but it's an important thing to consider. It might not be causing your child's lack of motivation, but it can exacerbate the behaviors that are there. And some of these are fairly easy to change.

A poor *fit with the environment* was a problem for Kenny, a fifth grader with ADHD who took medication for his symptoms of impulsivity and hyperactivity. The medication affected his appetite, and while his mother tried to get him to eat a good breakfast before he took his medication in the morning, there often wasn't enough time. The medication was working at its peak around his class's early lunchtime of 11:15, meaning that Kenny was pretty attentive but not very hungry. Unfortunately, his school didn't allow eating other than at lunchtime. So, when his appetite started to increase around 1:00, he started to feel sick with hunger pangs. By 2:00 P.M. Kenny was having trouble concentrating because he was cranky from not having eaten. When his dad picked him up from school at 3:30, he was angry and belligerent. His blood sugar was low, and he reacted with out-of-control behavior. He started to sound like a kid who couldn't care less—a kid who didn't "care about school," thought the medication was "ruining his life," and was "over-hungry" so that even the food that was offered to him wasn't very appealing. The home and school environments were not a great match for what Kenny needed. At home, he needed more time in the morning so that he could eat a good breakfast. That meant he needed to go to bed earlier at night. At school, there needed to be some flexibility so that Kenny could eat when he became hungry. This little bit of attention to

> *Can you tweak the environment so your child is in a better position to feel motivated?*

Kenny's goodness of fit made a very big difference in his ability to succeed at school. He came to school not hungry. The medication worked well, and with a snack in the afternoon he arrived home calm and nourished.

A *poor fit with the people in her environment* was a problem for Athena and her mother, Khadijah. Khadijah was an active, social mom who enjoyed parties and gatherings. When she wasn't at a get-together, she was outside— biking, playing tennis, hiking—begging Athena to go with her. Athena was a bit of a bookworm who enjoyed quiet activities. She had a tough time in large groups of people and was slow to warm up. Khadijah was often frus- trated and angry that Athena "didn't want to go anywhere," and the more demanding Khadijah became, the less eager Athena was to change. A few things needed to occur in this situation. First, Khadijah had to understand the child she had and not the one she thought she would have, which she assumed would be a carbon copy of her. This led to Khadijah having more realistic expectations. In talking with Athena, it became clear that she didn't want to be antisocial—she just couldn't handle her mom's constant need for social contact. Second, Athena did have some trouble with social anxiety that could benefit from supportive therapy. In addition, Khadijah started approaching these situations with more empathy and let Athena be Athena. They discussed their goals and expecta- tions and selected situations and activities that "fit" for both of them—like taking a yoga class together instead of a 20-mile bike ride on Saturday mornings.

> *Are there ways to create a better fit with your child by modifying your expectations for the child you have?*

CREATING AN ENVIRONMENT THAT IS A GOOD FIT FOR YOUR CHILD

The benefits of creating a home that is a better fit for your child can be particularly important for a kid who doesn't care. You avoid some of the never-ending battles over what you expect versus what they're capable of doing. You become more empathic and respectful, which typically builds trust—and helps kids learn to be more respectful toward you. Creating an environment that includes people who are in sync with your child is a proven way of supporting a child's self-esteem. The goal isn't for your child to become the kind of person who expects the environment to cater to her. The goal is to help your child recognize and put herself into situations and relationships that are a better fit for her as she moves into adulthood.

Here are more specific tips for *creating an environment geared for the child you have:*

* *Know your child's temperament and your own and identify how and where they don't fit together.* Sometimes knowing—and embracing—that we have a child who is temperamentally different from us can help relieve the stress of thinking that we're "bad" parents. Or worse—that we have a "bad" child.

* *Plan where your child might have specific problems* and brainstorm strategies (with them if you can) that will make it easier for them to behave.

* *Assess how well the environments fit your child's temperament.* School and home are the biggest areas, but places like afterschool care, Grandma's house, different home routines when parents live in separate places, can be a source of stress.

* *Consider the effect of your temperament on your child.* How do you typically react? Are you slow to anger? Or too quick? How do your reactions change the outcome of their behaviors?

* *If you know there are certain things that stress your child out,* decide which things are worth letting go. For example, if your child gets stressed in crowded places, don't force her to go to large sporting events or crowded malls during the holidays. It's a small thing, but to kids it can represent something much bigger—the fact that you understand and empathize with them.

* *Be aware of the language you use to describe your child* and replace some of the negative labels with positive ones.

* *Help your child think about ways he can fit better in all environments and help him pick environments that are a better fit.* This is one of the hallmarks of

a well-functioning adult—knowing ourselves and where we are most comfortable. That doesn't mean we avoid places that are uncomfortable. That's part of life. It means spending most of our time in places that fit who we are. It means thinking about what would make things better when we must be in environments that aren't a good fit for us.

Being in sync with your child is not the same as being just like your child.

Parental Stress and How It Can Interfere with Raising the Child You Have

All parents get stressed. There is no way around it. Stress in and of itself is not good or bad. It just *is*. It's the way we deal with stress that is the problem. My goal here isn't to help you fix every stress in your life. (There are some good books that can help with that, and you can find some of them at the end of this book.) My goal here is to point out that your own stress might be contributing to your child's tendency to be unmotivated. I know what you're thinking—"If I didn't have a kid like this, I wouldn't be so stressed." There is research to back you up on this, but that doesn't mean there's nothing you can do about it.

Let's first take a look at what we mean when we talk about stress. Stressors or stressful events fall into three categories:

• *Normal stressors*, like the day-to-day hassles of traffic or too much homework, or changes that occur when a child leaves for college or starts a new school. We can't avoid these types of stresses, and in fact some of them, like a new sibling or a move into a bigger house in a different neighborhood, are good. When people say, "Don't sweat the small stuff," they're usually talking about the normal stressors that often come with good things, like a busy life and growing kids, though we all know following this advice can be hard to do.

• *Unpredictable, often sudden stressors*. These are the big stressors that occur when someone becomes ill, is in an accident, loses a job, or experiences an event like a hurricane or fire. They don't always have to be quite this catastrophic. Sometimes an unpredictable stressor can be as simple as Grandma needing to stay with the family for six weeks after her knee replacement, but no one predicted that a simple act of kindness would change everyone's routines and make life chaotic.

• *Chronic stressors.* These are the stressors that occur and don't get better with time. In fact, sometimes they become worse with time. They're typically difficult to change. If you've got a child with a learning, emotional, or attentional difference, it's likely you and your child have experienced some level of stress with this. If your child has received good supportive services, you'll experience much less stress than will a family with a child who has had insufficient support, but there is chronic worry and stress nonetheless.

If you've got an unmotivated child, you're likely feeling stressed. If, on top of that, you've had unpredictable, sudden stressors (which nearly every family had during the 2020–2022 COVID-19 pandemic), you're even more vulnerable to feeling overwhelmed.

It's important to examine your level of stress, because when you're tense and worried, it tends to spill over into your child-rearing. You might become less affectionate and less responsive to what your child needs. This can leave you feeling guilty and more stressed. When parents are stressed, kids find a way to cope. Some kids become super-achievers. Others become aggressive. Still others become emotionally numb and "check out." However, when you help your child cope with stressful experiences, either by directly helping them or modeling adaptive coping skills when you're stressed, your child's ability to cope and be resilient is enhanced. If your major stress is your child, it's okay to tell him—"When you don't seem to want to do anything but sit in your room, I feel stressed"—but you can't stop there. You've got to then open up the discussion to him—"I can't imagine how you must feel"—and then listen and show him how you intend to cope with this stress, *yours and his*, by supporting him, finding the right help, keeping an eye toward the future. The diagram on page 146 can be a helpful reminder.

One thing to keep in mind. If you're thinking you're doing the right thing by holding in your stress and not letting anyone see it, you're not

Responding to Stress Step by Step

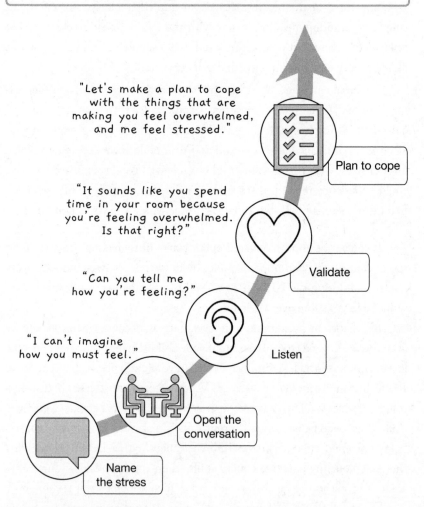

"Let's make a plan to cope with the things that are making you feel overwhelmed, and me feel stressed."

Plan to cope

"It sounds like you spend time in your room because you're feeling overwhelmed. Is that right?"

Validate

"Can you tell me how you're feeling?"

"I can't imagine how you must feel."

Listen

Open the conversation

Name the stress

"When you don't seem to want to do anything but sit in your room, I feel stressed."

fooling anyone. A recent study from Washington State University looked at families during the COVID-19 stay-at-home measures. They found that when parents tried to hide their emotions, children had a physical stress reaction that indicated they knew their parents weren't okay. When you say "I'm fine," kids know you're not and they are less likely to reach out to you if they are stressed or in need. We tend to tell kids "Everything is going to be okay," but it's more important that we honor our feelings and those of our kids. We need to give ourselves permission to be stressed and use those feelings to figure out how to reduce the stress in our lives. The way you react to stress provides your child with the model they will use in their lives; see the sidebar on page 148 for suggestions for coping with your own stress.

I hope this chapter has helped you better understand the complex interactions between your expectations and your child's behaviors. In the next chapter, we'll take a look at how parent behaviors (often well-intentioned ones!) can contribute to the problems of unmotivated kids. Before then, here's a review of some of the things discussed in this chapter to get you thinking, talking, and doing.

THINK, TALK, DO

 What to Think About

- What kinds of expectations did you have for your child when he was born? How have they changed since you first dreamed of having a baby?

- What helped you become more independent as a child? Is there anything from your own life that could be applied or shared with your child?

- What do you expect your child to be doing next year? In five years? In ten?

Coping with Your Own Stress

This is not meant to be an extensive list of how to cope with stress. If you are experiencing chronic stress, you might benefit from the support of an expert. There are resources in Chapter 12 that can help. What follows below are some general guidelines that have been found to be very effective in reducing stress in families:

- *Bring down the conflict.* "Okay," you might be thinking "it's the conflict that's making me stressed!" But conflict is often something we can change. For example, kids whose parents have divorced are not more or less stressed than kids whose parents did not divorce. What makes the difference is the level of conflict in the home. If parents divorce and they are able to resolve difficulties and keep conflicts to a minimum, their kids have the same outcomes as kids whose parents are living together peacefully. On the other hand, divorced parents and nondivorced parents who have high conflict in their relationships have similar rates of stress in the family. Thus, if there is any way to reduce the level of conflict in your family—between partners, extended family, neighbors—it's to your and your child's benefit to do it.

- *Keep to a daily routine.* It's often suggested that kids handle stress better when they know what to expect. Adults also handle stress better when they know the schedule and when things happen as expected. Simplify your life and keep to a daily routine that includes predictable and healthy sleeping and eating times.

- *Cut out anything you don't need to do.* Seriously. Do it.

- *Keep in touch with family and friends who are supportive.* The support of others is one of the biggest protective factors against stress, along with . . .

- *Exercise.* And it doesn't need to be much; a 30-minute walk four times a week is associated with all sorts of physical and psychological benefits.

- *Reach out for help.* Therapy, parenting groups, supportive family and friends, becoming more informed about your child's individual needs—all can help you process and relieve some of the stressors in your life.

- What do you imagine when you see your child as an adult who is your age?

- What are some of the stressors in your life? Which stressors are manageable and infrequent and which ones are chronic and difficult to manage? How many unpredictable stressors have you had to cope with in the last two to three years?

What to Talk About

- Ask your child where she sees herself in the next year, the next five years. What does she want to be when she grows up?

- Ask your child to tell you what he thinks *you* want him to be when he grows up. Talk about how that compares to the question above.

- Come up with a list of things that stress your child out. You might be surprised by the answers. Spend some time talking about environments that might be a better fit or ways to cope better.

What to Do

- Change the way you comment on your child's future—use their own hopes and dreams rather than your own.

- Write down the list of things that stress your child out (after the discussion you've had above). Make your own list too and, when appropriate, share your list with your child. Come up with a plan to change the things that can be changed.

- Find ways to keep in touch with family and friends who are supportive.

EIGHT

Adjusting Your Parenting Style to Fit the Child You Have

There are many ways to parent, and no single approach causes a child to look like he couldn't care less. This chapter will introduce you to the most common parenting styles and will take a deep dive into where many parents think it all leads—the college process. I really hope this chapter doesn't come off sounding like parent blaming. That's not my intention, nor would it be accurate. Parental behaviors occur in today's complicated social environment. I tend to think that in today's social-media-driven world, parenting styles and behaviors are at least partially created by the image-conscious society in which we live. We are hyperaware of what others are doing, and we don't want our child to be left out. Our best intentions cause some kids to say "Leave me out of all of this."

The field of psychology acknowledges at least four types of parenting styles—*authoritarian, authoritative, permissive,* and *uninvolved.* (See the sidebar on the facing page.) Of the four, authoritative is one most parents aspire to. It's associated with better outcomes, such as happiness, success, and better decision making in children. But even authoritative parents have unmotivated kids. Other things such as temperament, the school environment, and the influence of a child's peer group (addressed in the rest of this book) also play a role. I've observed parents who were once authoritative become authoritarian or permissive. The stress of having a child who couldn't care less caused them to be more of a strict disciplinarian or throw

Parenting Styles

- *Authoritarian* parents are the "because I said so" kind of parents. They believe kids should be seen and not heard and follow the rules without exception. The focus is on obedience, not on negotiating and compromise. This parenting style can cause kids who don't care to lock horns with their parents in battles that neither side can win. Sometimes having an unmotivated child will cause parents to become more authoritarian. This change is rarely effective.

- *Authoritative* parents spend a lot of time creating and maintaining positive relationships with their children. They have rules and consequences for misbehaving but explain the reasons behind the rules and empathize with their children. There is no question that they (and not the child) are in charge, but they allow their kids the opportunities to make decisions and take responsibility. This is the best parenting style for most kids, but when you have a child who couldn't care less, even the most authoritative parents will find themselves out of patience.

- *Permissive* parents are the kind of parents who make rules but never enforce them. They're the "kids will be kids" kind of parents who can often be more of a friend to their children than a parent. Kids in these households sometimes exhibit more behavior problems because they don't appreciate authority or rules. This parenting style is a bad combination for a child who doesn't care as it doesn't help her become more motivated.

- *Uninvolved parents* are ones who are, as the term would indicate, not involved much in their child's life. They tend to have few rules and don't devote much time or energy to parenting. Sometimes uninvolved parents are neglectful, but it's not always intentional. Uninvolved parents can be ones with mental health issues, substance abuse problems, or a severe medical issue. Parents who are uninvolved can cause a child not to care about much of anything. I usually find there is trauma involved somewhere in the family history. It can reach back into the parents' own histories or come in the form of a recent death of one parent, causing the parent who is left to check out due to grief. In these cases, helping the children who are struggling will almost always need to involve treatment for the parents, who are also suffering.

up their hands and become completely permissive. It's a good idea to reflect on where you fall on the spectrum of parenting styles, knowing that few of us fit neatly into a single category. Your style might have changed as a reaction to your child's current behavior. Or it may have needed to change and didn't.

Popular culture has added to these categories of parenting, and one of these might be familiar to you—*helicopter parents*. Helicopter parents are similar to authoritative parents. They most likely started out as authoritative parents. But then they became much more involved in their child's life. They are the parents who superimpose their own goals on their child. They pay too much attention to their child's activities, schoolwork, and social lives. They ensure their kids get the right coach on the second-grade soccer team and call professors when their young adults get a poor grade in college. They hover over their child's development like a helicopter. They *overparent* and tend to be *perfectionistic*. They *hate to see their child fail* and *conflate their own success with their child's*.

Most parents, except for the truly permissive ones, will find themselves being a helicopter parent from time to time. In my experience, most kids who don't care have at least one parent who displays helicopter parenting traits. I'm not at all saying that being a helicopter parent *caused* a child to become unmotivated or apathetic. It may work the other way around—kids who have certain temperaments might make parents develop a "hovering" style. Regardless of whether it preceded or was the result of having a child who couldn't care less, these kids tend to react very poorly to having a hovering, perfectionistic parent who is anxious about their success. Some kids can tolerate having a helicopter parent. Others can't, and many of those kids will start to look like a child who doesn't care.

> *Helicopter parenting can be caused by parental anxiety, perfectionism, and other factors, but whatever the cause, it can have various consequences for a child's level of motivation.*

Research has shown that anxiety might be an important underlying factor in the tendency toward helicopter parenting. Mothers who think the world is more dangerous tend to control their children's behavior more rigidly, maybe because they see the possibility of any failure as dangerous to their children. Other studies have shown that overparenting tends to be driven by *parent* needs rather than what the *child* needs. In that case, becoming clearer about what you want versus what your child wants might help you become less likely to overparent. Overparenting doesn't happen in a vacuum. Parenting in a pressure-filled world and other aspects of the environment—like worries about your child's peer group or the presence of a learning difference—can contribute to becoming a helicopter parent. Regardless of the reason, helicopter parenting is associated with negative outcomes such as these:

- Overparenting tends to give kids the message that you're proud of them only when they succeed, and you're terrified of their failing. As a result, kids believe that failure is to be avoided at all costs. Some kids literally avoid it entirely by not engaging in much of anything.

- Children of overinvolved parents are more likely to endorse feelings of entitlement because they think the level of involvement from their parents is what they deserve or require.

- Parent overinvolvement is associated with children who rely on extrinsic motivation (like grades and rewards) yet who have low self-efficacy (or the belief they have the capacity to control their behavior and motivation). This is an anxiety-ridden bind for kids. They need external rewards, yet don't believe they have the ability within themselves to achieve their goals.

You might be thinking right about now, "Okay, I get this is bad, but you don't understand. If I don't watch my child like a hawk, he would get even less done! Overparenting isn't a choice for me. In fact, he needs more oversight, not less!" I can completely understand where those thoughts come from. And you're right. Your child doesn't need less involvement from you. But he needs a different kind of involvement or mindset, not more of the same. In the next chapter, I'll talk about goal setting and how that is a better way to motivate children while feeling connected to them. Goal setting requires parents to set aside their tendencies to hover. The sidebar below provides some guidance in finding your way out of overparenting. But there's one thing to discuss before we explore goal-setting, and it's possibly the major cause of overparenting—*the college process.*

Finding a Way Out of Overparenting

Dr. Michael Ungar, a psychologist who specializes in resilience and parenting, suggests the following:

- *Reflect on your own childhood* and think about what helped you become more independent. In my practice, parents often say, "What worked for me was _____," and when I ask them, "Did you tell your child about that?" or "Have you tried that with your child?" they often hadn't even considered it. Our kids are a reflection of us, and what worked for us might work well for them too.

- *Think about what motivates your children,* particularly in their anxious, avoidant, or couldn't-care-less behaviors. You've heard this throughout the book, but it's worth repeating. Engage with your child about what messages they are hearing from you.

- *Find ways for your child to safely become independent*—from summer camp, to chores, to a part-time job.

In addition, I would add:

- *Be aware of the difference between being "involved" and "smothering."* Show interest and give support, but don't take away the ability your child has to "light" his own fire by snuffing it out with your interference. Don't "pile on logs" when what's necessary is a spark and air to fuel the flames (more about this on pages 155–157).

- *Get comfortable with logical consequences.* "You don't understand. If I don't help her finish her homework, she'll fail," parents will say to me. "Then she might have to experience failure," I'll tell them. "It's going to hurt—you and her. But you are giving her the ability to be responsible for herself—something most kids want."

Don't Be a Helicopter; Be a Fire Starter

I find that most parents who have a kid who couldn't care less eventually give up or hover excessively. Many alternate between the two, which can make life pretty miserable. I'd like you to think about a different model, using what you've learned thus far in the book. By now, I hope you've given some thought to your child's *aptitudes, pleasures,* and the things he likes to do, or *practice.* The ideal place to be is in the intersection of those three areas (to refresh your memory, see the Venn diagram on page 36). Use that information, along with the thinking you've done to answer the questions in the diagram below. In the middle of this triangle is the desire or "fire" that

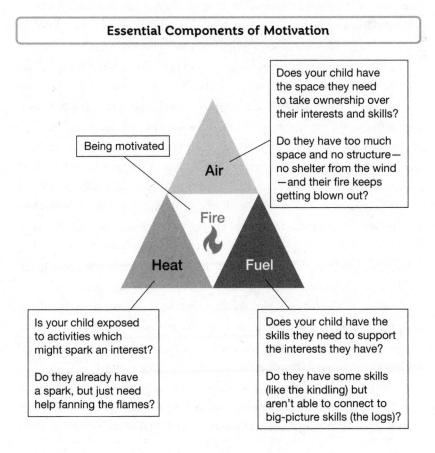

Essential Components of Motivation

Being motivated

Air

Does your child have the space they need to take ownership over their interests and skills?

Do they have too much space and no structure—no shelter from the wind—and their fire keeps getting blown out?

Fire

Heat

Fuel

Is your child exposed to activities which might spark an interest?

Do they already have a spark, but just need help fanning the flames?

Does your child have the skills they need to support the interests they have?

Do they have some skills (like the kindling) but aren't able to connect to big-picture skills (the logs)?

motivates a child. Fire demands at least three things—air, fuel, and a spark (heat). That's where you come in. Think of yourself as a firestarter, just not the Drew Barrymore variety. Imagine fire in its most wonderful form—a campfire on a cool June evening in the mountains or a fireplace in a warm cozy house. Both of these take a lot of tending, but once they're adequately started they take on a brilliant life of their own.

If we use fire tending as a metaphor for parenting, you need to think about three things—giving your child the *air* or space they need to learn about themselves—to find the right amount of structure that works for them. To have room to make mistakes. But they need the *fuel* or tools to be able to be effective. Those tools include lifelong "large" skills like fluent reading as well as smaller ones like studying for a math test. Finally, they need the *heat* or sparks that allow them to find a passion. Kids find this when they're exposed to interesting ideas and teachers and when they are surrounded by adults and peers who are excited about learning.

Many parents begin parenting by naturally doing the things in this picture. They surround their babies with lots of interesting toys. They give them room to fail as they're learning to run and speak. They structure their days with meals, naps, and bedtimes. They are the managers of their children's lives. Good parents are effective managers (or to use the fire analogy, fire tenders)—they find information, make contacts, help structure choices, and provide guidance. In infancy, this involves things like taking your child to the pediatrician and arranging childcare. In early childhood, it involves things like selecting the right preschool. In middle and late childhood, it involves setting rules for mealtimes, self-care, and appropriately helping with homework. Effective monitoring is very important in adolescence, but it can be difficult to manage for many families. The typical adolescent's push for autonomy can catch lots of parents off-guard. Most parents know it will get rough but can't imagine just how strong an adolescent's desires will be to spend time with peers or how intensely they can show their parents a need for independence—to be someone separate from the family.

When things go wrong, they often come to a head in adolescence, though the frustrations and anxiety usually start much earlier. Somewhere in this process of managing and tending, things have gone awry. A child wasn't given enough space. No one approved of the areas of life that gave him a spark. He didn't have the big or the small skills he needed to be successful. This happens for a lot of different reasons, but my sense is that for a lot of families the process is colored by a need and pressure to achieve. It can cause parents to hover, to disapprove of a child's choices, and to focus on developing the wrong skills. This "need to achieve" is nearly universally thought to require a college education. A lot of the

> *A child's "fire" can be extinguished by lack of exposure to what sparks interest, too little space to fan the flame, and/or too few skills to keep a strong fire burning.*

managerial work of parenting is geared with this in mind, and most parents aren't even aware that it's happening, and happening at an early age.

College Admission: Holy Grail and Fire Killer

I'm pretty sure that you want your child to go to college. I don't have a drone over your house recording your conversations. I am unable to read your mind. But I am pretty convinced of my assumption. "My child will go to a four-year college" is considered the Holy Grail of parenting a young adult. We've been told that it is indispensable to economic success and a fulfilling career. I'm pretty sure that you want your child to go to college because the idea that college is the key to prosperity is a point of view held by nearly every demographic group in the United States. It's not just college-educated or upper-income parents who expect their kids to go to college. Nearly *all* parents do.

IS COLLEGE THE RIGHT PATH FOR YOUR CHILD?

Bobby's mom was one of those parents. She called me one day in March in a panic. "I saw you speak at a conference," she said. "Will you evaluate my 18-year-old son? He's graduating from high school in two months. He's not ready for college, and I don't know how to make sure he's prepared. We decided that he could take next year off so he could catch up, but I don't know how to catch him up. He never studies and shows interest in nothing but the hardware store where he works on the weekend. Maybe if you could evaluate him and find what is wrong, you can tell me how to get him into college."

I wanted to help Bobby. In fact, everyone did. Even Bobby. The problem, though, wasn't that Bobby needed another evaluation. He'd had an evaluation of some sort almost every year or two since first grade. He had ADHD and a language disorder that made it hard to express himself, especially when he was nervous. The small group of friends he had from the neighborhood were all planning on attending college in the fall. Bobby's mother thought he was doomed to a meaningless life without a college education and felt embarrassed that her son was planning to take a year off. She was already fretting about high school graduation and the shame that she'd feel when someone inevitably asked her where Bobby was going in the fall.

"What will people think of us? I don't want to even make eye contact with other parents," she said. "He's the only kid I know who's not planning to go to college in the fall. I don't know what will become of him. I've failed as a parent, and I know he's disappointed in himself too."

I told Bobby's mom that a big evaluation wasn't what was needed. Instead, Bobby and his mom needed to find another way for Bobby to become an adult that didn't involve college. This was going to take some work because Bobby's mom, like the parents of all the other kids in Bobby's class, had been planning for her child's college education since he was very young. Some parents had been saving money in a college fund. Other families had grandparents who were ready to pay for college. Still others were prepared to mortgage the house or go into debt for the opportunity for their child to go to school. Going to college was the culmination of being a good 21st-century parent.

In contrast to Bobby are the kids who are desperate to go—or at least to get into—a good college. They sacrifice their free time and social lives so that they can get into a top school. Between these achievers and Bobby are the kids in the middle. The ones who are almost like Bobby but who stumble toward college, their parents filling out the applications. They don't want to go, but they do. At least for a year or two. In all these cases, college was the end of the yellow brick road of childhood. But like Dorothy in *The Wizard of Oz*, many find there's not much waiting behind the curtain except for a lot of smoke and mirrors. And debt. It can be a big disappointment for many of them.

HOW THE DRIVE TO GET INTO COLLEGE CAN STALL MOTIVATION

The drive to get into college might be one of the biggest underlying causes for lack of motivation in many kids who couldn't care less. And I'm not just talking about high school students. Kindergarten has become the new first grade, with an emphasis on academic outcomes and less time spent on play, social interactions, and exploration. This emphasis didn't come from the drive to make kids better hairstylists or house painters. It came from the idea that strong academics will lead to stronger students who will one day be ready for college. Yes, the drive to get in starts early, and bright kids who don't like what they see on the horizon will start to check out as early as middle school. Aspirations for success force kids to do everything at the peak level of performance. In the mad rush to achieve are kids who have a mad rush to relax and use substances. The higher-achieving kids are frequently caught in a cycle of achieving and relaxing—working without much sleep during the week and partying hard on the weekends. The kids who aren't interested in school are caught in a cycle of never achieving. Many kids vape, and use other substances, as a way to feel some sense of control.

Driven kids lose motivation when they pursue activities and achievements whose only meaning for them is whether it will help them get into some prestigious college.

This isn't just an upper-class problem. The pressure to perform pools in affluent neighborhoods, but it doesn't stop there. The fierce competition for college admissions among the upper and upper middle classes raises the bar for all students who hope to get in. Research has indicated that although external circumstances may differ, most students across demographic strata feel unsupported, stressed, and inundated with what constitutes success. They know it's not just a small house and a happy life. Instead, it's a life filled with Instagram-worthy vacations, designer homes, and a job that will change the world. For that you need AP classes and the right college. But before you can get there, there's the idea that you need the right math class in sixth grade, the special sport talent by fourth grade, and the right preschool to start you on your way.

Kids who don't feel driven to get into college can end up caught in a cycle of not achieving, and they may use substances to feel some sense of control.

From my vantage point, the drive to get into college leaves a lot of kids behind, and many of those kids start to not care. The kids who buy into it participate in activities that don't interest them. They see their peers as competition. Their parents spend money on tutoring and test preparation that doesn't build meaningful knowledge. Admission to an elite college is something that defines them—or it doesn't. Some of those kids are crushed because they worked very hard and didn't get what they thought they deserved. Others just decided not to care much about it at all. For those who get in, there is often disillusionment. "Is this what I worked so hard for?" Or "If I'd worked harder, I wouldn't be here."

College doesn't seem as much fun as it was when I was a student. Some of that might be a good thing. The drinking age was still 18 then (I'm showing my age here), and there were lots of parties with alcohol, many of them sponsored by the college. Now many colleges are alcohol free. Some have a "one strike and you're out" policy. If you're caught drinking in the dorms or attending a party, it might result in being asked to leave—permanently. This is a tough policy for adolescents who are prone to making mistakes and who need space to make them. Increased rates of depression and anxiety in college students—along with dropout rates of 40% from four-year schools and close to 70% from community colleges—would attest to the fact that something isn't working.

But it's worth it, right? My child will make more money and have a better lifestyle?

Not exactly. The data on that aren't as solid as you might think. A brief from the Brookings Institution in 2013 showed that while a college degree can be a good thing—about $570,000 of extra income over a lifetime for a bachelor's degree—those figures are averages. They apply only to college graduates, and they don't consider the school type and the choice of major. They also don't take into account the debilitating debt that changes the entire life path of a student or family. Starting a first job—or entering retirement (as is the case for some parents who assume their child's debt)—with $250,000 or more of debt can lead to a life of unrealized expectations.

> *We need to listen when kids say they don't want to go to college, because our efforts to get them in anyway often don't pay off—they lead to dropping out, depression, and hopelessness.*

I spent the first 20 years of my career as a psychologist doing everything I could to make sure kids with learning disabilities, ADHD, and other developmental differences could get into college. I helped them get the right accommodations throughout elementary and high school. This made a very positive difference for hundreds, if not thousands, of kids. But it didn't work for all of them. If I had met Bobby 15 years ago, I would have mounted a full-court press to find a way to get him into college. Over the years, I found that too many Bobbys (and Olivias too) dropped out of school after a few semesters, depressed because college wasn't for them and hopeless because they (and often their parents) thought there was nothing left. I don't want to give the impression that all these kids had learning differences or that kids with learning differences are less able to make it through college. That's not the case at all. The problem was that I wasn't listening closely enough to what the kids were saying. Sometimes it was easy to hear what they were saying—"My parents think I should go to college, but I don't want to go." Their parents would arrive in my office saying "What's wrong with her? Who doesn't want to go to college?" Other times it was more difficult. Those were the kids who would parrot what their parents said. When asked what they wanted to do after high school, they'd say "I guess college." Their actions—skipping classes, not turning in homework, arriving late every day for first period—told a different story. They didn't want to go to college, but no one—including me—could imagine a different path after high school.

This is not to say that kids who couldn't care less shouldn't go to college. Sometimes kids who don't care in high school do very well once they leave for college. There could be dozens of reasons why. Maybe it was the high school or social environment that caused them to check out. Maybe they just needed to grow up. However, they probably showed *some* interest in college, even if they showed little interest in other things. If your child is one of those, you can use the college process to motivate them now. Most often, these kids are ones who are still getting good grades, or at least showing up for class. They might hate their school, their peers, or their home life. They might have been shunned by the best friend they'd had since first grade or checked out when their parents announced they were getting divorced and Dad started dating a woman half his age. When working with kids like these, I will first confirm that indeed they do want to go to college. I'll identify what is getting in their way. Frequently it's not something they can change, but at least acknowledging it is helpful. And then I'll tell them, "Okay, so what we need to do is figure out how to get you from today to your first day of college. Let's figure out a plan."

IS YOUR CHILD READY?

So how do you know who is ready and who isn't? Here are some questions to ask yourself:

• *Is your child excited about the prospect of college?* Lots of kids are stressed about the college process, but there should be excitement too. Not wanting to go look at colleges, never talking about it, or not wanting to get out of the car when you take your child on a college tour is a clear sign they are not interested in attending.

• *Did your child fill out the application by herself?* Many kids will need a little help with applications. They might need help editing their essays or staying somewhat organized, but for the most part they should be able to complete the application independently. This is my number-one question to ask parents. If the answer is no, and especially if it's "Are you kidding? The kid doesn't even know his password to the Common Application," I can almost guarantee that child will be back home within two years. There are exceptions to every rule, but there are very few to this one.

• *Did your child get good grades?* If she's not getting good grades in high school, she's not going to miraculously get better grades in an even tougher environment.

• *Did your child attend class regularly?* One of the clearest signals kids give that they aren't ready for college, especially during the late junior and senior years of high school, is to stop going to class. If your child is not going to class, with you yelling at him to get out of bed in the morning, he will most likely not independently start to go to classes in college.

• *Do they have an idea of what they want to study?* The career your child wants at age 17 is not necessarily the career they will eventually have. About 80% of college students change their major at least once. But a child who is ready for college will have some ideas. She might think she wants to major in French because she loved her high school French teacher and a family vacation to Paris but end up majoring in nursing. He might want to study economics because his uncle is an economist but switch to math and become a middle school math teacher. But both examples have one thing in common—a student who wants to study *something*. Students who are ready for college are interested in areas of study or want a career that requires a college degree. When children don't have either interest or a career goal that includes college, it doesn't mean they are not college material. It means that their interests don't line up with what college has to offer or that they are not ready to make those kinds of choices. Some kids might have a pat answer as to why they're going to college, ranging from "It's where my mom went" to "I love the football at University of Michigan." Those might not be the most mature reasons to go to college, but they're at least some type of reason. Kids who couldn't care less tend to not even have "pat" answers when asked why they should go to college. They might just shrug, or they might say it's something they actually *don't* want to do. Rarely do I find them faking an interest in college when none exists. Rather than making that an issue that becomes a battlefield, look at it from the other direction: "You're not interested in going to college, so let's come up with a different plan. Where should we start?"

For information on alternatives to college, see the sidebar on page 165.

WHAT ABOUT BOBBY?

You might be wondering what happened to Bobby. Perhaps you remember that he loved working at the hardware store. He especially enjoyed helping people with their construction projects—assisting them in finding the right paint, nails, and tools. One of his customers, a carpenter, had offered to hire and train him. When Bobby had originally brought up this idea to his mom, she immediately dismissed it. In my work with them, we used the Parenting APP—*aptitude, pleasure, and practice*—to see if this would be a good fit for him. Bobby already knew it would. He loved working with his hands. He loved the idea of a pay increase. He felt confident he could learn the necessary skills. His mom was able to see this as a valid—and even exciting—choice.

I shared Bobby's story and the problems with the quest for college not because I think you should let go of your dreams of a college education for your child, but because I think you should be open to other ideas when they're appropriate. Many kids who don't care are successful in college, and many kids with perfect academic records aren't. The message is to remember who your child is—their interests, their temperament, how they spend their

What Are the Alternatives to College?

The idea that there is one path for every student is, in my opinion, one of the biggest contributing factors in youth depression, anxiety, and the tendency to not care much about anything. We've got to let go of this notion. There are some great resources on this topic at the end of this book, but here are some alternatives to get you started:

- *Get a job.* Some kids who couldn't care less when they're at school do very well transitioning right into a career. It gives them a purpose, a structure, and immediate success. One student athlete I knew started working at the reception desk at a gym. Within six months, he began training as a fitness instructor. He was making a very good income before his high school classmates finished college. I've heard similar stories from students who worked their way up from the bottom of the ladder in fairly short periods of time in the fields of real estate, cosmetology, hair styling, restaurants, and software design, just to name a few.

- *Get an apprenticeship.* Some apprenticeships are more competitive than college, but they're worth applying for if your child has interest in a job in a field such as construction, manufacturing, health care, cosmetology, or transportation, where on-the-job experience is key.

- *Go to community college.* This is a great halfway step for the student who wants to go to college but isn't sure what she wants to do or for one who would like to work and take a few classes to see what college is like.

- *Coding* is a field that is attractive to students who would prefer to go right into the work field. Coding bootcamps are short (usually less than six months) and often immediately lead to good job offers.

- *Think outside the box.* This thinking needs to start by listening to your child. Listen to what they want and then brainstorm what they might enjoy doing. I've watched kids become a hairstylist, work as a skipper on a private yacht, become a pilot, join the military, get training in HVAC, work as a sales representative, manage a medical office, work on a farm, and become a chef. And that's just for starters. All these jobs have potential for growth. Sometimes a college degree is required for advancement, and it's not uncommon for the kids who didn't want to go to college at age 17 to enjoy the college experience at 28. Their degrees are often then paid for or subsidized by their employer.

time, and what they are good at doing—and to understand how you can best "fit in" to help them realize their dreams.

Trying to Be a "Good Enough" Parent Is Good Enough

Parents who raise the child they have are *good enough parents*. They are not perfect parents. They make mistakes, are inconsistent, and might not always have aspirations and expectations that are perfectly in line with their child. If you've read this chapter and thought, "Well, I completely blew it! I've been trying to parent a different kid than I have," you're not alone. If you're in the middle of *striving* to be a good enough parent, then you're already there. Parents who are striving to be "good enough" have expectations that are consistent with their child's age and abilities. They have the capacity to empathize with their child's point of view. Every parent can learn how to do this, and it's something that even the best parents (if there is such a thing) need to continue to work toward. I'm hoping that this chapter and the ones preceding it have given you ways to better understand your child. The next section of the book, *Keys to Helping Your Child Care More*, gets more specific about how to use the knowledge you've gained about your child to set appropriate goals and how the right mindset will keep the process positive and resilient.

THINK, TALK, DO

What to Think About

- What are the experiences you had in your childhood that you hope your child will have? What experiences would you like her to avoid having?

- What are your aspirations about college for your child? Have you always had these goals? How would you feel if your child didn't attend college right after high school?

- What kind of parental style do you tend to have? If you've got more than one child, does it differ depending on the child? Has it changed over time?

- To assess college readiness, think about your answers to these questions:

  - Does your child get good grades?
  - Does your child consistently (always) attend class?
  - Does your child know what she wants to study?
  - Does your child talk about where they'd like to attend college and why?
  - Is your child capable of filling out the application independently?

What to Talk About

Use these questions to start a conversation with your child about their hopes for the future:

- Are you excited about the prospect of college? What excites you/doesn't excite you about it? Do you know what you want to study?

- Imagine yourself at age 15, 20, 30, Grandma's age. What kinds of things can you imagine doing? Why do you want to achieve those things?

- Imagine a perfect day as an adult. What would that day look like?

Answer these questions for yourself and your child. What do you see yourself doing in 10 years? What hopes do you have for your child? Convey this information in a way that makes it clear that your hopes are not their hopes and that you have dreams of your own for yourself. This helps to make clear the boundaries between your future and theirs.

✎ What to Do

Use the activity on page 169 as a way to pull all of the information in the last few chapters together. (If you need more space to fill this out, you can download and print a copy from *www.guilford.com/braaten4-forms*.) The lines leading from the "You are here" circle are only an example of possible outcomes. Use your answers to make some hypotheses about where you are and where you'd like to be.

Write down the expectations you have about your child's future and separately have your child write down their expectations. Do the same for your and their temperament and interests. See where they match and where they don't. Are there areas where there seems to be little compromise? Are there extra stressors that are making it difficult to meet or even think about meeting goals/expectations? Identify them and talk about how they might be decreased or eliminated.

On page 170 is an example for Bobby.

Pulling It All Together Activity

Expectations

What I say to my child about their future:	What my child says about their future:	Stress:

$\times$ $\times$

Goodness of fit

My temperament and interests:	My child's temperament and interests:

=

You are here

- Helicopter parenting?
- Quest for college?
- Perfectionism?

Pulling It All Together: Bobby

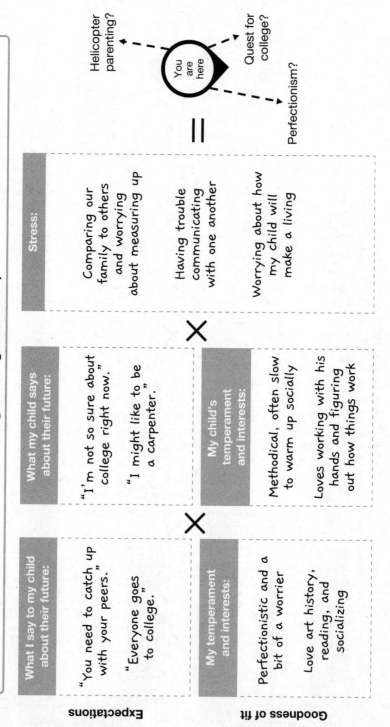

Expectations

What I say to my child about their future:
"You need to catch up with your peers."
"Everyone goes to college."

My temperament and interests:
Perfectionistic and a bit of a worrier
Love art history, reading, and socializing

Goodness of fit

×

What my child says about their future:
"I'm not so sure about college right now."
"I might like to be a carpenter."

My child's temperament and interests:
Methodical, often slow to warm up socially
Loves working with his hands and figuring out how things work

×

Stress:
Comparing our family to others and worrying about measuring up
Having trouble communicating with one another
Worrying about how my child will make a living

=

Helicopter parenting?

Quest for college?

Perfectionism?

You are here

PART III

Keys to Helping Your Child Care More

NINE

Set Goals That You Can Both Get Behind

Kids, especially kids who couldn't care less, often have difficulty identifying the endgame. "What's the goal? What's the point in all of this?" they'll ask when they're discouraged or overwhelmed. Parents on the other hand have lots of goals in mind. In the last chapter we discussed the pros and cons of having college education as a goal. But there are other (seemingly very good) goals that parents have that can sometimes get in the way of setting real, achievable goals that help kids move from not caring to feeling successful. As I said earlier in this book, one of the most frequent "goals" if not the *most* frequent that I hear from parents is "I want my child to be happy." This is particularly true for parents of kids who couldn't care less, because they often don't seem very happy and parents understandably worry that their child will never break out of this cycle.

It's easy to understand why parents want their kids to be happy. People who describe themselves as happy are more likely to be in successful relationships. They tend to spend more time helping others. They're generally thought to be more likable. They even sleep better. You might think that a chapter on goal setting might include a goal about how to be happier. But happiness isn't a goal. It's the *result* of good goals. It is an outcome rather than the goal itself. The first part of this book was about identifying things— the APP: *aptitude, pleasure,* and *practice*—that your child does well, enjoys doing, and spends time doing. The second part of the book gave you some ideas about how things like temperament or expectations can get in the way of helping kids stay in the APP zone. But identifying the factors and obstacles in your child's APP is only the beginning. We have to use this information to set reasonable goals.

Happiness is not a goal. It is the outcome of reaching good goals.

Kids who couldn't care less are very often unhappy kids without goals. If they do have goals, the goals aren't often shared by the people who love them. Identifying appropriate goals and using them to motivate behavior and find meaning in life is one of the most important ways to help your child.

What Defines an Effective Goal?

Goals is a term we use a lot. But we might not completely understand how to apply goals effectively. Here's some basic information to get the conversation started (questions to ask are presented in the sidebar on page 175):

- Goals need to be *chosen and not dictated.* Children need to choose their goals independently. When you hear your child talking about an interest, approach it as an invitation, rather than something your child "must" do. Kids don't often use the word *goal* except in a vague way, like "I want to play for the New York Yankees" or "I want to be a fire fighter." See the sidebar on page 175 for more information on how to help kids generate ideas for goals.

- Goals need to be *clear and specific.* It can be helpful to write them down. You might be thinking that there is no way that your 13-year-old is going to write down a goal for the school year, but if you approach it knowing his APPs, and giving him the opportunity to define what he wants, writing it down can be a simple next step. You can even use the excuse that you're writing it down so that *you* don't forget.

- Goals needs to be framed *positively*, not as a threat but as a challenge they can meet. (See the A in APP to make sure they have the ability. If

Questions for Opening a Conversation about Goal Setting

Goal setting isn't an event but a process. It's a skill that kids (and adults too!) need to constantly be using and revising. Some good questions to keep in mind when trying to get your child to think about goals include the following:

- What makes you happy?

- What do you look forward to?

- What makes you feel excited?

- What things are hard for you, but you like doing them anyway?

- Who are people you admire? Why do you admire them?

- What do you hope to accomplish this school year . . . this season . . . this week . . . in your history class?

These kinds of questions need to be part of a family's "vocabulary." I find that parents often think they know what makes their child feel excited or what the child wants to accomplish in a given school year, but have never actually asked their child. Ask even more than you think is necessary.

not, help them frame the goal in a way they can achieve.) The steps toward reaching the goal need to be *clear* and *not too far in the distant future*. If it's so far away that you can't imagine the steps, then it's not a real goal. For example, "I want to get all A's at the end of the year" from a B/C student who struggles with reading would not be a good goal. Picking a couple of subjects in which to excel and a short time period (the first month of school) is a better option.

- Goals need to be *mastery focused* in that the goal should build on a skill your child already has some familiarity with.

• Goals *aren't just a one-time thing.* You should come back to the goals again and again. Reflect on what worked. Revise when necessary. Try again. It's okay to let go of goals—we don't accomplish everything we set out to do—but when we let them go, we should be aware of the process. Indeed, being flexible *is* part of the process. Revising one's goals is the key to success.

Choosing Goals That Are Clear, Specific, and Developmentally Appropriate

I've said this before and it's worth saying again—*kids who couldn't care less are kids without achievable goals.* Setting goals, planning how to achieve those goals, and monitoring the success toward those goals are incredibly important aspects of children's and adolescents' development and achievement. Without them, kids might feel like they're adrift in the world. When kids are lucky, they have an adult in their life who points them in the direction of developing appropriate goals—like the art teacher who opens up the world of drawing, a great coach, or the owner of the ice cream store where they worked over the summer. Mentors like these are important because *they give kids goals.* They say "You've got talent in art" or "The customers really like you. You've really got a head for business." This is the place to start when talking about setting goals with your child. Depending on the age of your child, you might not ever use the word *goal.* If you have an eight-year-old who doesn't seem to like much of anything, you can start the conversation by saying "Let's think about how you'd like to spend your free time this school year." With a 14-year-old who is having difficulty in school, you could start the conversation with "How can we change the course of this semester?" or "What would make you most happy this semester?" These types of conversations help kids choose what they want. It can make them more motivated when they know exactly what they

To get a goal-setting conversation started, you don't even have to use the word goal; *you can ask what the child wants to do for the summer or semester or for available free time.*

are working toward and more self-confident when they see progress in something that before might have seemed pointless.

The SMART acronym has been used for decades within the business world to guide goal setting. *SMART* means that goals have to be *specific, measurable, achievable, relevant, and time-based*. These ideas have been shown to be effective for kids too. Nonspecific goals such as *"I want to be a CEO"* are not very useful, though I find these types of goals are frequently reinforced by parents, like the parents of a boy I'll call Teddy.

SMART GOALS THAT WORK

"He really seems like an entrepreneur," Teddy's parents told me about their son. He was 12 at the time. "A lot of them like Bill Gates and Zuckerberg didn't finish school, so I wanted to cut him some slack with his grades. Not everybody can be a great student, but he used to at least try. Now that he's in middle school, he doesn't seem to want to do anything. He's so far behind, and there's nothing we can do about it. He's never going to be a CEO the way he's going."

I met Teddy in November of his eighth-grade year. He explained to me that his seventh-grade year was hard. "My best friend, Will, moved to Florida in February," he said. "And then when baseball season started, I broke my arm and couldn't play." Teddy went on to tell me that after Will moved he felt lonely and it was tough to find new kids to hang out with. Baseball season started, and he began to feel hopeful again until he fell off his bike and broke his arm. A summer that he'd hoped to spend swimming at camp was spent playing video games and watching everyone else do the things he wanted to do. He started eighth grade feeling fairly depressed.

"I want to do okay in school," Teddy said. "My parents think I don't care, but I do. I just don't want to do what they want me to do. And they think I can catch up on homework, but there is no way I can."

Taken together, the last nine months had been an isolating and confusing time for Teddy. He found it hard to complete his work for many reasons. As soon as he sat down to do his homework (on the days that he actually *did* sit down), a feeling of dread would wash over him. He'd plan to study his Spanish vocabulary or finish his algebra homework, but then found himself inevitably scrolling through TikTok or bingeing on YouTube videos. By the time his parents were telling him he needed to get to sleep, he'd have accomplished nothing other than feeling overwhelmed or, as he described it, feeling like "I'm a loser."

Teddy's depression made it hard for him to care about much of anything. When we're depressed, it's hard to find motivation. Compounding the depression, Teddy had started to feel anxious, which was making it hard for him to sleep. The lack of sleep was making it hard for him to pay attention, and this cycle of depression/anxiety/lack of sleep/poor attention was leading to even deeper feelings of depression.

The process of goal setting with Teddy started with my asking him, "So, Teddy, if I had the power to give you one wish, what would you wish for right now?"

"I just want to feel better," he said.

We spent some time talking about what that meant, because using the SMART acronym, the goal has to first be specific. As we talked it became clear that Teddy wanted to feel less depressed and less anxious, so "To feel less depressed and anxious" became our first goal. It fit all of the SMART categories. Not only was it *specific*, but it could also be *measured*. It was *achievable*, very *relevant* to Teddy, and could be *time-bound*. To tackle this goal, Teddy agreed to participate in cognitive-behavioral therapy for four months. During that time, he'd talk with his therapist about what was working and what wasn't and would review his progress every two weeks. He was also open to trying medication for his depression if therapy didn't work to treat his symptoms as quickly as he wanted.

Once Teddy was able to articulate his number-one goal, I asked him for two more. "Okay, Teddy," I said. "You've now got three wishes. The first one is to feel less depressed and anxious. What would the other two be? And one of them can't be more wishes!"

It surprised Teddy's parents that it was so easy for him to come up with the other two—to do better in school and to start playing sports again. It didn't surprise me. Kids often know exactly what they want. His parents, like most parents who are anxious and frustrated by a kid who couldn't care less, were afraid the answers would be something they wouldn't like. But the goals he had were goals they could easily get behind, though it might take some time to identify and complete the tasks needed to complete these goals. It was fairly easy to come up with a list of tasks to help Teddy feel less depressed and to get more involved in sports. The tasks involved things like finding an appropriate therapist, working out at the gym with his dad, and trying out for the basketball team.

> *We sometimes assume that unmotivated kids don't have any idea what they want, but kids often know exactly what they want.*

Doing better in school was a bit more complicated. Okay, in all honesty, it's a lot tougher, in part because "doing better in school" isn't a specific goal. I started the conversation about this by asking "What do you need to do to feel like you're doing better in school?"

Teddy looked down at the ground. "I don't know," he said. "I don't think I can. It's impossible to catch up."

"Let's find out if it is," I said. Together we made a list of all of Teddy's outstanding assignments. His list looked like this:

- Turn in all algebra homework, some of which was already done but not yet turned in
- Read *The Nightmare Thief* for English class
- Make a three-minute film for Spanish class
- Retake his history test
- Write up two experiments from science class

As we looked at the list, Teddy had two opposing thoughts. On one hand, this seemed insurmountable. On the other hand, it looked like less than he had imagined. Before he'd written this down, he felt a lot of anxiety, but he wasn't quite sure exactly what he was anxious about. Now he could see it. While it was going to take some work, it was a finite list.

Teddy and I then talked about where he should begin. We talked about when he would have time to complete these tasks and whether it would help him to talk to his teachers about what he'd been struggling with. We wrote a plan of action for each item, figured out the order in which he would tackle each one, and a specific date when the action should be completed. Teddy decided to talk to his teachers and found it helped. His history teacher allowed him to retake his history test orally, which left Teddy feeling less pressured. His English teacher allowed him to listen to *The Nightmare Thief* as an audiobook. Teddy also got a tutor to help him organize and complete his outstanding homework. There was no magic pill that helped Teddy go from a student who couldn't care less to one who cared more, but his—and his parents'—perseverance paid off. Teddy caught up and finished the school year having met his goals. In the process of getting back on track, Teddy and his parents realized that the traditional public high school might not be the best fit for him. They explored alternative private and public options, and Teddy found a charter high school that was a better match for his learning style and interests. (See Chapter 10 for more information about when switching schools can be helpful.)

The keys to Teddy's success hinged on the fact that the goals were broken down into clear, specific action plans that included answers to questions such as: "What is it that needs to be accomplished?" "Why is this goal important?" "Who needs to be involved in helping Teddy accomplish the goal?" "What are the resources that he needs?" If the goals seemed unrealistic, Teddy was encouraged to tweak them or make new ones. Clear time limits were set as to when the goal would be accomplished so that there was a deadline to focus on and work toward. When goals weren't met, time was spent trying to understand why. When goals *were* accomplished, they were

When a Child Is Too Depressed to Care

Many things can lead to depression, such as loss of friends, stressors such as parental divorce, and medical issues. When a child is significantly depressed, the first goal should be to seek treatment for the depression. In fact, severely depressed individuals are often too depressed to set goals.

celebrated, and new hopes and dreams were discussed (and made into new goals).

Engaging Kids in Goal Setting

Teddy's journey makes goal setting sound so easy—pick a goal, plan how to reach it, and do it. If only it was as easy as I made it sound! When kids are depressed and anxious, or stuck in a not-caring attitude, many things can get in the way of their setting and completing goals. But there are some ways to engage your child and set them up for success. Here are some things to keep in mind:

• *Ask your child if she thinks she can do it.* If the answer is no, the goal is not reachable—*even if you think your child should have answered yes.* I once had a parent of a fourth grader say to me that his child was going to major in "pencil nib" because all his child ever did was stare at the eraser nib of his pencil when it was time to start a writing assignment. This is often a child who doesn't think he can do what is asked of him or doesn't know how. He needs a goal that is broken down into manageable steps. Let's say that the child staring at the top of the pencil is given an assignment like "Write a two-paragraph essay on your favorite TV character." That might sound fairly easy for some kids, but for this student it's too broad a concept. He needs to start this assignment with "Let's talk about some of your favorite TV characters." Followed by "Do you have a favorite?" and "Why is that character your favorite?" Though this is a small task, you can generalize it into bigger goals. Notice that I didn't start with "Who is your favorite TV character?" That might be too much pressure for some kids, who might not know how to pick a favorite. For any task you're asking your child to do, make sure it feels like a step he can take. If it's too big, break it down. Ask her about the steps she'd take to make it happen. Do those feel manageable? If not, break those down to even smaller steps.

• *Be realistic about how long it will take.* I learned (or in this case relearned) a lot of lessons during the pandemic. Quite a few of them had to do with time. One of the many "time" lessons I learned was the result of my sitting on Zoom for large portions of the day. I developed a nagging neck pain that developed into shoulder pain and then eventually numbness down my arm. When I finally (after much *time* had passed) realized that the pain and numbness was getting worse, I went to Colin, a physical therapist. He gave me some exercises to do and told me it might take some time to feel better. I was discouraged after one week that not too much had changed. I was overly optimistic that I could change something that was months in the making and was incredibly discouraged that I didn't get complete, immediate relief right away *after I did all the right things*—for seven days. My physical therapist gave me an idea of how long it *might* take to get relief (six to eight weeks), but I chose to stick with how long I thought it "should" take. Be aware of this trap when you're working on habits and behaviors that are hard to break and were long in the making. It's also a good idea to remember that old habits can come back. When the pain in my shoulder came back after months of being pain free, I became incredibly discouraged again. My physical therapist assured me that this was normal, but all I could think was "I already met this goal. I did the treatment, so I shouldn't have to deal with this again!" Don't get demoralized when these things happen. They're normal and to be expected.

  • *Timing is everything*—not only with regard to how long it will take, but also in keeping track of time. Many kids who couldn't care less have poor *time perception*—they can't estimate how much time has passed or discriminate between different time periods. It's hard for them to tell whether 10 minutes have passed by or 40. This can make it hard to stick with time-specific goals. Help your child better learn a sense of time by keeping track of it for him. Don't only remind him that he has 10 minutes, or two days, left before he has to complete a project. Let him know that he's been *working* for 10 minutes, or four days, so that he begins to develop an internal sense of time. Using things like electronic calendars, notifications, and alarms are great as reminders. But they assume that kids understand the concept of time. We spend a lot of time teaching kids *time management* skills. But we can't manage something we don't understand.

Setting Goals That You *Don't* Want to Happen

An important exercise when goal setting can involve talking about goals that you *don't* want to happen. You might find that your goals and your child's are particularly aligned when it comes to bad outcomes. I find that parents are quite good about knowing what they *don't* want to happen: "I don't want my child to be held back in school." "I don't want my child to fail algebra because she didn't turn in her homework." But kids have only a vague notion of what they don't want to happen. That vagueness can lead to a sense of anxiety and fear that only slows them down. Ask your child about the number-one goal (or the top three) he *doesn't* want to happen. He might say something like "I don't want to fail chemistry." "I don't want Cheryl to break up with me before the prom." "I don't want my parents to always be mad at me." While you can't help what happens with Cheryl, you might agree that you also don't want to see your child fail chemistry or to spend the year angry at him. Talking about goals you *don't* want to reach can be a way of *reaching out* to your child. (And as a side note, when it comes to the relationship with Cheryl, file this information away so that when the breakup inevitably happens, you'll realize how devastating it is—and use this information to help your child readjust his goals.)

• *Build in accountability.* If we know someone else knows our plans, we're more likely to complete them. Kids who have trouble completing goals often avoid accountability because they're afraid of failure. They might bristle at the thought of having to be accountable because it never ended well for them. Help them understand that this time it's different. It's not a matter of a thumbs up or down but a matter of monitoring their success and helping them if they haven't achieved what they set out to do.

• *Don't forget rewards!* We do things because they lead to positive outcomes—otherwise known as *rewards*. While I'll feel a sense of accomplishment when I finish this book—which can be rewarding in and of itself—I wouldn't be doing it without the reward that comes when someone buys the

book (*and thank you in advance!*). Big rewards and small rewards were important to me. Build these things into your child's life. Small things like outdoor play, snacks, socializing, social media, and large things like going on a
special trip at the end of a semes-
ter need to be part of the fabric of
your child's life. One caveat:
Don't choose rewards that are
addictive. Social media (or food
or video games or TV) time is a
reward for some but not for others. Choose your child's rewards
carefully.

> *Kids who couldn't care less often
> need to sharpen their perception
> of time, but this means not just
> reminding them of how much time
> is left before a deadline but also
> pointing out how much time they
> just spent working on a task.*

There are many applications and resources for helping your child
choose goals at different ages, and we've included many of them in the
resources in Chapter 12.

The Goals Have Been Made—*Now What?*

New Year's resolutions are frequently broken because they are made but not
monitored. A goal without consistent, conscious follow-up is just a wish. It's
an easy trap to fall into, particularly if you've got a child who couldn't care
less. When kids who didn't seem to care finally have goals similar to those of
their parents, everyone breathes a big sigh of relief. In fact, getting everyone
on the same page feels so different—so much less angry and anxiety provok-
ing—that many families think they've already reached the goal.

Renee was an 11-year-old who stopped doing her homework when she
started sixth grade. There were many reasons for this, including an undiagnosed learning disorder in math and problems with organization. "Thanks
for helping us figure out why Renee was having so much trouble," her parents told me. I gave them a long list of recommendations, such as tutoring
and support at school, that Renee needed to be successful. But her parents
didn't want to use those recommendations to create specific goals. They

were so relieved that Renee's problems weren't occurring because she was depressed, lacking intelligence, or, in her mother's words "a budding juvenile delinquent like my sister," that they didn't immediately take the next steps, like getting an IEP at school that included math tutoring. When they called me six months later because "Renee isn't any better," they admitted they hadn't shared my test results with her school, afraid they'd stigmatize her. They needed some counseling as to why these goals were important for Renee, as well as information on what to do once the goals were enacted.

THE IMPORTANCE OF MONITORING PROGRESS TOWARD GOALS

Goals, once embraced, need to be monitored. How do you do that? First, *make sure the goals are written down somewhere* accessible. Goals that are written down have a much greater probability of being accomplished. They also serve to help you remember exactly what the goals are. Second, *give lots of feedback*. Praise your child's success and effort. There will be roadblocks and failures. Be honest about them when you see them. Ask them why they think things didn't work out as they'd planned. Talk to them about your own failures that might be similar. Help them figure out how to change their goals.

In addition, you want to build in a sense of autonomy. Teach your child to ask for help only after he's tried some solutions on his own. Don't rescue them by fixing things. Provide emotional and structural support. If their solutions sound like they're not going to fix the problem, brainstorm new ones. Gently push them toward solutions that will guarantee a greater chance of success. Finally, build in scaffolding. When your child is consistently successful at something with your help, start removing the help so that they feel a great sense of accomplishment and responsibility.

> *Working toward goals should build your child's sense of autonomy, so ask why your child thinks she hit a glitch, share your own failures, and support her rather than leaping to the rescue.*

What Does It All Mean? Finding One's Purpose

In William Damon's book *The Path to Purpose,* he talks about how successful identity development is a long-term process that involves reflection. It sometimes means postponing decisions or saying no to things that others think are important but that you know aren't important to you. The idea of *purpose* is a crucial part of identity development. Finding a purpose involves answering questions such as "*Why* am I doing this?" and "*Why* does it matter?" and "*Why* is this important to me, to the people I care about, or to the world beyond me?" It's the *why* we do what we do—and it means accomplishing something that contributes not just to our own development but to others as well. Setting, achieving, and readjusting goals can help kids find their purpose.

In writing his book about finding purpose in our lives, Damon asked adolescents and young adults, ages 12 to 22, questions like the ones above. Only 20% of them had a clear vision of where they wanted to go in life, what they wanted to achieve, and why. Another 20% expressed having no aspirations, and some of those said they didn't see any reason to have any aspirations at all (I have a feeling many of these kids had a couldn't-care-less attitude). The 60% in the middle had done some purposeful activities, like volunteering or talking with their guidance counselors about the future, but then didn't really have any ideas about what their goals were or how to achieve them if they did. They did the things everyone told them they were supposed to do, but it didn't lead to their finding what *their* purpose was.

Part of the problem is that parents and kids too often focus on short-term goals, like tomorrow's science test or getting the right number of hours to fulfill their volunteer requirements for graduation, but they don't spend enough time talking about the future and what they desire. You might have a child who says things like "Who cares about studying? No one's going to look at my grades when I get a job." This is a child who doesn't understand the connection between studying hard and getting good grades. Kids like this will often ask questions like "What's the point?" which is another way of saying "What's the purpose?" When parents try to make the connection for them, it's often something like "Without good grades, you'll never amount to anything!" instead of "People who care about getting good grades want to continue in school. Good grades lead to better opportunities. Look, if you don't want the kinds of opportunities that better grades lead to—if you don't want to go to college or apply to a private high school—we can talk about that. But then we also need to talk about what bad grades lead to, too." Kids who say they don't want to get good grades usually *do* want better grades, but either they don't know how to do so (sometimes that can be due to a learning disability) or they're trying to tell you that they don't necessarily want the kinds of opportunities that getting good grades provide. If you're a kid who doesn't like school and good grades lead to more school, getting bad grades is one way of telling adults that one of your goals would *not* be more school. Talking to kids about bigger, broader life goals and desires is a much better way to resolve conflicts such as these. It can also help them develop a positive identity. Adults can't answer the question "What is my life's purpose?" for a child, but we can provide guidance, feedback, and opportunities where they can experience success. Kids need environments where they can be inspired and not demoralized. Adults need to spend more time listening to what kids want and less time assuming we know. This doesn't mean we let them do whatever they want. It means providing guidance, feedback, and opportunities that are in line with their aspirations. Good questions to get the conversation started include ones like these:

- What kinds of things are important to you?

- Why are they important? What makes you care about them?

- Imagine yourself at age 15, 20, 30. What kinds of things do you think you'll have achieved?

- Why do you want to achieve those things?

- Imagine a perfect day as an adult. What would that day look like?

- What does it mean to be a happy person? A person with good character?

- Imagine you're Grandma's age. What kinds of things would you want people to say about you?

- What are the sorts of things you admire in other people? Do you want to be like them? Why?

Motivation endures when a child understands the connection between an effort and an outcome and when goals can be connected to long-term meaning and purpose.

Answers to these questions can provide a starting point for setting goals as well as help your child find the meaning in those goals. You can participate in this discussion as it relates to *your* goals too. Kids aren't the only ones who need to focus

Goals Can Be Set at Any Age

Although I've used examples of middle and high school students in this chapter, goals aren't just for teens. In fact, the lack of goals in early childhood is one of the reasons some adolescents have no sense of what a goal is or why they're important. Kids of any age can learn to set goals. Goals for younger kids can be:

- *Educational:* Learning long division, going to the library twice a month, reading a picture book to your little sister, learning a new skill (like how to bake cookies), taking piano lessons

- *Safety and health:* Always using sunscreen (something that can be difficult for kids with sensory sensitivities), wearing a seatbelt, getting more sleep

- *Nutritional:* Trying a new food once a week, eating less junk food, learning to "cook" a meal in the microwave

- *Fitness:* Playing outside for 30 minutes a few times a week, taking a bike ride with Mom, taking swimming lessons

- *Relational:* Spending more time with grandparents (or keeping in touch if they live far away), asking the new kid at school for a playdate

Why Are My Child's Goals So Grandiose?

Although much of this chapter is about kids who couldn't care less having too few goals, some have goals that are far too lofty, and many kids have both—only a few goals, all of which are unattainable. What do I mean by unattainable? These are goals like "I want to be a rock star . . . a CEO by age 20 . . . a professional football player . . . an Influencer . . . a TikTok star . . . "

Some parents, like Teddy's, fuel these goals a bit, but many kids come up with them on their own. We can blame social media, the fact that we value money over strengths like humility, or call it the *American Idol* syndrome. We value money and fame in our society, and money and fame aren't always linked to talent. What is a parent to do?

- *Know your child's aptitudes and use that knowledge to lead discussions about unrealistic goals.* You don't want to squash your child's dreams, particularly if they are somewhat realistic. At the same time, it's okay to point out when they have unrealistic goals. You just want to make sure you first . . .

- *Know why your child has that goal.* What is it about that lifestyle or choice that makes them want to aspire to obtain it?

- *Talk about why you think the goal(s) are unrealistic.* Are there statistics that you can quote that help make your point? If so, use them.

- *Make the goal tangible.* Being a billionaire is not a goal. It's the result of many goals. Help your child understand this concept. Help them create a plan for achieving the goal.

on the future. Adults can benefit from making goals, and you can provide a powerful example of how goal setting is a lifelong habit. Keep a family journal where everyone in the family answers these questions at different points in the year, such as the start and end of every school year. Keeping our eyes focused on the long-term goals—knowing that most of us want a life as an adult with a clear sense of identity and purpose—helps us make and appreciate the short-term goals. It's okay if your child's answers change over time.

Kids may want to pursue one career one month and another the next. They might dress or act one way (even to the point of changing their pronouns) one year and do something different the next. This experimentation is the way that kids (particularly adolescents) find out where they fit in the world. The important role for parents and teachers is to keep listening and focusing on the future, while challenging kids as to whether their behaviors are leading them where they want to go and into the person they want to become.

Teddy Revisited

Earlier in the chapter I introduced you to a boy named Teddy. By the end of his eighth-grade year Teddy was a huge success story. Much of this success was due to Teddy, but his parents and teachers played a big role too. At the end of eighth grade I was asked to join him and his parents and teachers for a planning meeting for high school. Things were going well until his parents started asking questions like "Why aren't you suggesting all AP classes for him next year?" and "Don't you think he'll stop trying if we don't push him in high school?" I started to worry that all the work we'd done helping Teddy learn to care more was going to be ruined within the first semester of high school. The teachers started getting a bit defensive about their recommendations for Teddy's ninth-grade courses.

"Doctor," Teddy's dad said, looking at me, "what do you think Teddy's capable of? You said he's got an intellect that's in the top 10% of kids his age. Shouldn't he be challenged?"

I took a deep breath and said, "Teddy has the capability to do anything he sets his mind to. *Could* he get all A's in AP classes in high school? If grades were based on intelligence, the answer would be yes. But why would he *want* to do it? Why would *anyone* want to do it? While there is the occasional student who really loves studying just for the sake of studying, Teddy hasn't shown us he's one of those students. He's got a lot more that interests him than just studying for AP classes. Most people—including really smart ones—pick one or two things they love and then choose to do their best in those areas. Teddy would be much better off picking a few classes—ones that he loves—where he can embrace the challenge rather than being challenged in everything and embracing very little."

A couple of teachers started applauding. His parents looked a little relieved.

"Could you tell this to the rest of the parents of kids in Teddy's class?" the guidance counselor asked.

We all laughed because we all knew we were a little bit of the problem. It's not just that parents put pressures on kids. Teachers do too. Psychologists like me ask for accommodations for kids like Teddy so that they can push themselves as hard as they'd like. These things aren't wrong. We all have Teddy's best interests in mind, but it's easy to overdo it. In years past, I'd been involved in meetings where teachers encouraged kids to take the hardest classes in high school, where parents insisted on putting their child in courses that were too difficult, or where I advocated for significant accommodations for kids who might have been better off in classes where they would feel more comfortable and autonomous.

In these cases we'd somehow lost sight of the child. Kids who have the highest self-esteem are those who perform competently in areas that are important to them. Thus, children and adolescents need to be encouraged to identify and value areas where they are capable. This sets them up for something called a "growth mindset"—a view where children believe their qualities can change and improve through their effort. A growth mindset is something that is often missing in kids who couldn't care less. It's hard to nurture this kind of mindset without the right kind of goals. Now that you've got some ideas about how to set goals, it's time to talk about using them to promote an attitude where a child starts to learn to care more. But before the next chapter, here are some things to think about, talk about, and do.

THINK, TALK, DO

 ### What to Think About

- What is the first goal you can remember having? Did you accomplish it? If so, how? If not, what happened?

- What practices do you use to move yourself toward goals? Would those practices work for your child? Why or why not?

- What goals do you have for your child? How realistic are they? How well do they mesh with your child's goals for himself?

💬 What to Talk About

- When talking about starting a goal:
  - What exactly is it that needs to be accomplished?
  - Why is this goal important?
  - Who needs to be involved in helping you accomplish the goal?
  - What are the resources that you need to accomplish this goal?
  - What kinds of skills will you need to achieve this goal?
  - How long do you think it will take to accomplish this goal?
  - How will you keep track of your progress?

- When talking about an ongoing goal:
  - Is there anything unexpected (good or bad) that could potentially happen while you're pursuing this goal?
  - Do you feel like you can accomplish the next step independently? If not, what help would you need?
  - What have you learned about yourself while pursuing this goal?

✏️ What to Do

- There are many books on goal setting for kids, some of which are listed in Chapter 12. They are filled with activities that can be used to help create individual, classroom, and family goals.

- Use these worksheets as a way to begin setting goals:
  - *https://inside.sou.edu/assets/socsci/Advising__Student_Success/Goal_ Setting/ica.SMARTGoalWorksheet.pdf*
  - *www.sandiego.edu/hr/documents/STAFFGoals-PerfPlanningGuide1.pdf*
  - *www.chemeketa.edu/media/content-assets/documents/pdf/students/ student-services/counseling/career-development-model/GoalSetting- Worksheet.pdf*

TEN

Stay Flexible to Keep Your Child Motivated

Pick up any good book on education or parenting these days and there's about a 90% chance you'll run across the term *growth mindset*. If you haven't heard the term, then you've probably heard some of the often-used phrases that for better or worse came out of the growth mindset movement—things like "praise the effort, not the child" or "I know math is hard for you, but you *tried*; that's what's important" or "Not everyone is good at science, but don't worry; you're good at other things." Understanding the concept of growth mindset and how to help your child use it in a flexible way to solve problems and make goals is an essential part of increasing motivation.

Growth and Fixed Mindsets

The term *growth mindset* was originally coined by psychologist and researcher Carol Dweck, who was interested in figuring out why some kids developed resiliency and others didn't. Her research stresses the importance of developing a *mindset*—the mental picture we develop for ourselves—focused on *growth*. According to Dr. Dweck, we can have one of two mindsets. The first type, a *fixed mindset*, is one where we believe our qualities, or *who we are*, are fixed in stone and cannot change. The second, a *growth mindset*, is one where we believe our qualities can change and improve through our efforts.

Having a fixed mindset can leave people feeling helpless—"What can I do about it? This is just who I am"—while a growth mindset sees challenges as opportunities: "If you only go through life doing stuff that's easy, you'll never learn anything that's hard or interesting."

Kids' mindsets influence whether they will be optimistic or pessimistic. Their mindsets shape their goals and affect their achievement and success in school and sports. When kids have more of a fixed mindset—when they think their abilities are set in stone—they tend to give up in the face of a challenge. When they are criticized or hit an obstacle, they often view it as proof that they indeed don't have the abilities they need to be successful. On the other hand, kids who have more of a growth mindset assume their talents and abilities can be developed. They believe that learning something new or sticking with something that's difficult is the way to get better at it. While they know kids can have special talents in sports or the arts or academics, they don't think that talent is the only thing that's important.

Mindsets begin to be formed as kids interact with parents, teachers, tutors, and coaches. It's complicated, because while kids are developing their own mindsets about themselves, the adults around them may have already become "fixed" on who they think that child will be. As you read this chapter, I want you to think about how adults in your child's life may influence your child's mindset through their speech and actions. For example, a third-grade teacher might already have a fixed mindset about certain kids in her new class because she's read the reports from the second-grade teacher. "Pamela is chatty, distractible, and doesn't seem to care much about reading" becomes "Pamela is the not-so-bright girl who cares more about her friends than schoolwork. Thus, I'm not going to push Pamela too hard in academics."

Mindsets and Kids Who Couldn't Care Less

When I first started thinking about why developing a growth mindset is important for kids who couldn't care less, my bias was that it was a black-and-white issue. Kids who don't care have a fixed mindset (one that goes something like "I can't do this") and are surrounded by adults who hold pretty fixed views about them (one that goes something like "He's just lazy, and come to think of it, he's always been like this"). I was wrong. While these sorts of fixed mindsets are definitely a piece of the puzzle, it's a much more complicated issue. See if one or more of these scenarios fit for you, because the solutions to the difficulties will differ:

• *You used to be a parent who had a growth mindset—one who thought your child was capable of being almost anything—and you've lost it.* If this is you, spend some time thinking about where it went wrong (the previous chapters might help you figure out whether it might have been the result of a bigger problem). That child you thought could do anything didn't disappear.

• *You have a growth mindset—you still think your child is capable of almost anything—but your child has a fixed mindset.* You might think the appropriate "fix" for this is to help your child develop a more flexible, growth mindset, but you first need to examine your mindset, or at least the way you show it. Do you say things like "You're so smart!" or "You've got more talent in your pinkie finger than the rest of us put together!"? Those are seemingly great things to say, but when we're down on ourselves, the last thing we want to hear is how we're not using our unrealized potential. In addition to examining your own behaviors, you'll want to explore the reasons your child *does* have a fixed mindset (Chapter 11 provides more information about what to do when you're really worried).

• *Your child seems to have been born this way.* There are parents who will say, "He's been difficult since the day we brought him home." As you might remember from Chapter 6, sometimes kids are born with difficult temperaments. If this is your family, it's going to take some work to uncover the strengths that are hidden in your child. Sometimes working with a therapist can help change the behavior patterns that typically occur in relationships like these.

• *You and your child have a growth mindset (or are at least striving to have one), but your child's school environment sees your child as "fixed."* If this is the primary cause for the not-caring attitude, addressing the problem means addressing the school environment, through developing or redesigning your child's IEP, helping the teacher become better informed about what your child needs, and advocating for your child. Sometimes it takes a change in school placement to replace this mindset (you'll read more about things to consider in changing a school placement later in this chapter).

Each one of these scenarios requires a different approach to changing the behaviors. These changes are going to take a bit of insight and then applying the things you've learned in other places in this book to supporting a growth mindset. In fact, when you've got a kid who doesn't seem to care about much of anything, I see the process more as one of developing a *flexible mindset.* One that rolls with the punches and is open to thinking about people in new ways. One that truly believes people are capable of change at any point in development.

Why Having a Flexible Mindset Is Essential to Caring More

The research on developing a growth mindset has been applied to individuals, businesses, and education. Kids and adults who believe their talent can be developed through hard work, mentoring, and learning things like better study skills are more likely to have a growth mindset. They tend to achieve more because they worry less about how they're doing and put more energy into what they're learning. When schools embrace a growth, or flexible, mindset, kids generally feel more empowered and committed. In contrast, in schools and companies where there is a fixed mindset, cheating and deception are more common. Good schools generally have a growth mindset approach, but sometimes schools with good students have more

Schools filled with good students can have the fixed idea that all students are smart, which can leave some students feeling like they'll never measure up.

of a fixed mindset than you might think. They can have the "fixed" idea that their students are smart, talented, and naturally built for success. This can lead to students thinking things like "Everyone at this school was born smart, and I don't measure up." It can lead parents to think that extra time on tests, instead of studying more effectively, is the answer to better scores on their child's SAT.

Kids with intellectual disabilities and learning disorders have higher rates of fixed mindset attitudes than do kids without learning challenges. When kids have both, they're more likely to also have emotional and behavioral issues. The good news is that the skills related to a growth mindset can be learned. Children who were diagnosed with depression and anxiety who received just a one-session growth mindset intervention were less depressed nine months later than were children who did not get the intervention. Kids with reading disabilities who participated in a reading intervention coupled with a growth mindset intervention outperformed children assigned to only the reading intervention.

Most people (and organizations) are normally a mix of fixed and flexible mindsets. As I've said before, kids who don't care tend to be stuck somewhere in the fixed zone, but the goal isn't to change their outlook completely; rather it's to help them become more flexible. Having a flexible mindset isn't about praising and rewarding a child's efforts (see more about the dangers of this below) so that they feel good about themselves just for trying. Outcomes matter. Kids know when an adult is heaping on false praise. When adults do this, motivation tends to decrease and the inflexible mindset gets stronger. Research on growth mindset has shown the importance of rewarding not just the process but the actual *progress, learning,* and *outcome.* Adults also need to emphasize *why* positive outcomes happen—by pointing out the importance of seeking help from others, trying new strategies, and learning from mistakes. The research shows that actively engaging in this process leads to positive outcomes.

Kids with fixed mindsets have particular difficulties when things go wrong. It can be something small, like a bad grade on a spelling test, or a big mistake, like showing up drunk to a school dance. A fixed mindset can make it impossible to get past the inevitable blunders and problems we encounter in life. If you think, "Well, this is who I am," it's hard to become anything else. This is particularly true for kids with learning and behavioral difficulties. They spend a lot of time being asked to "hurry up" or "do better" or "try harder." Because trying harder is rarely the solution, and especially if no other solutions are presented, mistakes can result in reinforcing the fixed ideas they have about themselves. This might lead them to *not* try new things or to *not* take risks that might lead to better outcomes.

Kids know when adults are showering them with false praise.

APPROPRIATE RISK TAKING

Schools that directly embody a growth mindset don't just have a mission statement posted on classroom walls. They encourage appropriate risk taking, with the knowledge that some risks won't work out. They reward students for important and useful lessons learned, even if students don't meet their goals. There is less of an emphasis on grades as an end goal and more on grades as a way to measure progress. Collaboration rather than competition is supported. These schools are committed to the growth of every student, not just in words but in actions, by having places where every student can achieve. Varied extracurricular activities, consistent feedback, and clear measuring of progress are all important.

MEASURING PROGRESS

One of the quickest ways to jumpstart a child with a fixed mindset is to begin to find ways to measure progress, starting with tasks and goals that are achievable. In addition, numerous studies have shown that interventions that provide students with scientific information about how the brain changes through challenge, failure, and subsequent learning help kids develop a more flexible mindset. For example, one study by Lisa Blackwell and her colleagues found that seventh-grade students who were given a growth mindset message (something like "Here's how your brain develops when you learn math") along with study-skills tutoring increased their math achievement later in the year compared to those students who received only study-skills tutoring. The key is to educate students on the fact that their effort makes a difference and to back it up with scientific evidence that learning something new actually changes the structure of their brains.

TRYING SOMETHING NEW

I'm guessing that your child is hesitant when trying something new. It's sort of embedded in the definition of a typical child who couldn't care less. But having a flexible mindset can help when transitioning to something new. It can help kids focus on what is in their control and can reduce the crippling fear that they will be stuck in their current state forever. It helps them become more confident about taking the initiative instead of becoming reactive or disengaged. But it's not enough to simply give them information on how the brain develops or to simply encourage them to keep trying. Teachers and parents need to help kids evaluate the strategies they are using. If a student keeps trying to study the same way and keeps failing, the goal is to encourage the student to try a new approach and to help the student understand when to take appropriate risks. Feedback is important. If you've got a kid who is completely disengaged, the place to start is by saying something like "Nothing has been working well, and we need to find a different way." Talk about his APPs, use them to generate some small goals, and then give lots of feedback about what is working and what isn't once you start to work toward those goals.

One important point: The goal of the flexible mindset is not to send the message that your child can, or should, persevere through every challenge or negative life situation. There are some situations—like bad teachers or chronic bullying—that are completely toxic and that no improvement in mindset can overcome. There are other situations—such as undiagnosed or untreated learning disabilities, depression, or anxiety—that can't be fixed with a better mindset and need to be treated with well-studied strategies and tools.

False Praise: Where Having a Flexible Mindset Can Go Wrong

This idea of growth mindset has been so popular that it's been a victim of its own success. At the beginning of this chapter, I noted that you might have heard or used phrases like "That's great! You really tried hard!" These sorts of phrases, while fine in small doses, in larger doses actually undermine a child's motivation. Well-intentioned adults, who read about how it's important to foster growth, misunderstood this as being similar to the idea of encouraging growth by saying "You can do it!" The idea of a growth mindset was actually developed as a counter to the "every child gets a participation trophy."

There's a lot of concern today that too many kids grow up receiving empty praise. I find that kids who couldn't care less often fall into one of two scenarios—they either don't get *any* praise *or* they've been given praise for performance that is mediocre or even poor. Sometimes the mediocre performance is the result of not having the right instruction. For example, Howard was a 12-year-old who had been diagnosed with dyslexia. He was an amiable kid who tended to roll with the punches and not complain. He never got the intensive reading instruction he needed so that he could read at the same level as his peers, but he had enough instruction to move along to the next grade. He'd gotten a lot of unmerited praise for "doing great!" and "I like how hard you worked this year!" in the hopes it would prop up his self-esteem. When his parents separated, Howard was in fifth grade and unable to keep up academically. Shuffling between his parents' two homes, frustrated at school, he began to look like a kid who just gave up completely. The false praise he'd heard in third grade didn't work anymore in fifth. Helping him develop a flexible mindset would have to include addressing the causes of his difficulties. He needed to be able to achieve and to measure his achievements. Straightforward teaching of reading skills resulted in increased achievement for Howard. When he knew what it would take to be a better reader—and when he was given the opportunity to learn those skills—his mindset changed. As he became a better student, his self-esteem improved. Like many kids, his self-esteem improved because he faced a problem and coped with it rather than avoiding it while being told he was doing fine.

In terms of praise, one important difference was that Howard's teachers and parents learned to praise the effort that led to the *outcome* or learning progress. They didn't just praise the fact that he was *trying* but tied the *trying* to the *outcome*. They helped him find different strategies when he was stuck. They showed him when it was important to ask for help. They stopped saying things like "Not everyone is good at reading. Don't worry, you're good at other things." Those statements had conveyed to Howard that reading was something that was "fixed" and that offered little possibility of change.

Praising the effort is fine as long as the trying is tied to the outcome.

With different messages he learned that reading ability actually was something that can change significantly with the right kind of teaching. He learned that good strategies, hard work, and consistency lead to better learning.

Motivating Students Who Have a Fixed Mindset

The development of mindsets can be seen in children as young as three or four years old. Research has demonstrated that the way a parent reacts to a child's failure is an important early influence on a child's mindset. When parents react to their children's failures as though they are negative—if they immediately try to rescue the child—kids begin to develop the idea that whatever they were attempting to do is important and that they can't do it. Parents are usually pretty good at avoiding this very early in development. For example, when kids are learning to walk, parents expect they will fall. A lot. Toddlers who are first learning to walk will naturally cry when they trip and bump their head on a coffee table. But the assumption is that this skill will develop. Parents don't pick children up and say "Not everyone is good at walking. You are good at talking!" while carrying them everywhere so they don't have a chance of once again bumping their head. They don't say "I like how you're trying to walk." They hold their hands, slowly letting go, then moving away and saying, "Come here! Keep going!" Beyond those early years, parental anxiety can more easily get in the way.

When toddlers fall while learning to walk, we don't say "Not everyone is good at walking—you're good at talking!" and then carry them around everywhere to prevent future falls. We teach them how to make progress at walking.

The way you handle your child's failures conveys a lot of information to a child about your own anxiety. Kids who couldn't care less have typically had a lot of failures. How have you reacted to these? Did you rush in to fix things? Get angry? Reassure your child? Do you act now like there is nothing that can be done? If you've answered yes to the last question, that's a sign that your thoughts about your child are pretty fixed. Here are the things parents say that indicate they might have a fixed mindset:

- "What will he even make of himself? He's never going to amount to anything if he's getting mostly C's in sixth grade."

- "Well, if she's not going to college, what could she ever do?"

- "Oh, he'll never be able to pass Spanish. He has enough trouble in English class!"

- "I can't imagine that she'll ever be successful . . . live alone . . . cook for herself . . . make it to work on time . . . be able to survive without me to remind her what she needs to do next."

Keep in mind that the vast majority of kids do learn to survive on their own without parents to remind them what they need to do next. When asked, "What do you think is the most important ingredient in kids becoming independent?" I usually answer, "They grow up." Trust that even the most difficult kids can grow into pretty wonderful

What is the most important ingredient in kids becoming independent? They grow up.

adults. In the meantime, here are some effective strategies you can use to enhance the process:

• *Use failures or setbacks as a way to enhance learning and understanding.* Even if you're at your wits' end right now, you can start by asking "Okay, what has all this been teaching us?" You can summarize for your child what the problem is—you all probably already know, but it's good to verbalize it, as it makes it less scary. It could be something like "Fourth grade isn't going so well. I'm anxious. You're not doing your homework. What can we learn from this? What should we do next?" Figure out the next step. Is it talking to the teacher? The school psychologist? Getting an evaluation? Letting your child know that you are "on it" helps them a lot. Things often get better once parents schedule an appointment with a psychologist for an evaluation or treatment (even before they arrive for the appointment). Scheduling the appointment lets a child know that this issue isn't fixed. Even posing the question "What do you think would be most helpful?" gives a child the information that they aren't stuck in this problem forever.

• *Be more matter-of-fact* in your use of praise. Sometimes kids who couldn't care less have parents (sometimes only one) who praise everything in the hopes that this will motivate them. Praise without a connection to something tangible is never a good motivator. Effusive praise is never convincing, especially when coming from a parent. On the other hand, you don't want to be too passive. Finding the middle ground is key, but it's one of the hardest places to find when you're a parent, and the middle ground won't be the same for each child. There are no "rules" to follow. Be a careful observer of the process.

• *Talk to your child about how the brain is "like a muscle" that needs to be exercised.* Working out at the gym leads to stronger muscles, weight loss, and better skills. The brain works the same way, except that the "gym" is spending time with books, learning new things, and exploring new ideas alone and with others.

When Changing a Fixed Mindset Requires a Change in School Placement

Parents of kids who couldn't care less are desperate and will frequently ask me whether a change in school placement might be what's necessary. My usual answer is "My bias is to keep the child where he is if possible, and if a move is necessary, we've got to make sure it's right." Changing schools is disruptive for kids, especially kids in grades 8 to 12. It's always better to deal with what you know than with what can possibly happen at a new place. That being said, if a child has been in the same situation since kindergarten—a situation that might include a lack of a peer group or being inappropriately "labeled"—and now as a sixth grader feels like he's still the same ineffective kindergarten student, it might be time for a change. A child who was labeled "the biter [the kid who bit other kids]" in preschool and "the hyperactive kid" in first grade and is surrounded by the same small group of parents and kids in sixth grade, can find it tough to be seen as someone different. However, I do think parents should explore every option with school staff before making a change, as there are no guarantees that a change in placement will lead to a real change in behavior. When a change in placement does *not* go as planned, it can be doubly disappointing for kids and parents and only serve to reinforce a fixed mindset. However, I have seen many kids benefit considerably from changing schools.

SIGNS THAT YOUR CHILD MAY NEED TO CHANGE SCHOOLS

When should a child switch schools? Look for the following signs:

- Your child is chronically unhappy and lacks an appropriate peer group (see below for more thoughts about this).
- They're not making progress academically, socially, or emotionally, or more importantly . . .
- They're regressing (this is probably the most important consideration).

If your child is sliding backward, a big course correction is usually indicated.

- You're worried your child is being bullied by other students or teachers and you're worried about their safety.

- The school doesn't meet your child's basic needs—the curriculum is too hard or too easy; there are no appropriate creative outlets or extracurricular activities; your child has a specific learning challenge that is not being addressed appropriately; your child is socially isolated.

Making a switch needs to be thoughtful and is a process that, when handled well, shows the value of a growth and flexible mindset. You want to make sure your child hears something like "I don't think the message you've been getting at school is correct" or "The school you're in now isn't allowing you the freedom to grow. Let's find a place that provides you with different opportunities." I've found that sometimes just *exploring* the public and private school options has a therapeutic effect on some kids and families. Options, even if you don't act on them, can have a way of settling anxiety. Occasionally, after a long search of other schools, parents come back to me and say, "He's going to stay where he is for now. Maybe we'll make a change at high school." Looking at other choices helped them better evaluate their current school placement and determine ways to make it better.

> *Sometimes just knowing other school options are available can ease anxiety about whether your child's current school is the right one.*

Factors to Take into Account When Considering a Change of Schools

But let's say that you're seriously considering making a change. What are some of the things to think through when making a switch?

● *Your child's feelings.* You want this change to be seen not as a failure but as a positive opportunity for growth. If you've deemed the transition absolutely necessary, to the best of your ability, make it a positive experience. Engage in goal setting—ask the child what she wants in her next school setting. Are there clubs or activities that can get her excited about the switch? Many times kids are really relieved to change schools, but it's difficult for them to express this to their parents, as it seems like a failure. If this is the case, give them the words: "Listen, I know it's hard to switch schools, but I want to find a way to make things better for you." If you're beginning the search, engage them by saying, "Let's just see if there are some other schools that might be a better match for the way you learn best."

● *Your child's friends.* If parents tell me that a child has a great peer group at school, I'm more hesitant to encourage them to make a change, especially if the student is already in middle or high school. The ability to maintain appropriate relationships is not easy, and a new school placement will make it more difficult to find those close relationships. Sometimes the child has given up because school became hard and there is an undiagnosed learning or attention problem that is making some aspects of school difficult (academics) and others not (social relationships). In that case, addressing the problem of the learning challenge is a better place to start than changing the school. On the other hand, if your child has no social relationships and you see little possibility that he can break into a new peer group (for example, he's been with the same group of kids for five years and no one has invited him to a birthday party), the social issues of changing schools are less of an issue. In fact, the absence of an appropriate peer group is one of the best reasons to make a change. Regardless, you want to make sure there is a plan for integrating your child into a new social milieu while helping them maintain existing relationships.

● *The new school environment*—teachers, curriculum, class size are all important factors. Make sure the curriculum is growth oriented, that there is enough staff to meet each child's needs, and that the qualifications of the teaching staff are appropriate.

● *Extracurricular activities*—if you've got a child who couldn't care less,

Switching schools is about more than a better academic environment. The potential for good social relationships is just as important.

you've likely got a child who doesn't participate much in extracurricular activities. Reassess your child's APP (what they're good at, what gives them pleasure, and what they tend to do). If you're making a change in schools, be absolutely certain that the new school offers opportunities for your child to explore his passions.

Ways to Develop a *Realistic* Mindset in Kids Who Couldn't Care Less

Developing a realistic mindset means putting into practice the other things we've explored in this book—things like identifying what gives your child pleasure, setting better goals, and understanding your child's temperament. These kinds of recommendations take time. In the meantime, you might feel frustrated that you're not doing enough. Luckily, there are things you can do immediately that can help to foster a growth mindset in your family. Here are some ideas:

• *Reframe what it means to fail.* Instead of asking your child, "What went well today?" try asking, "What didn't go well for you this week?" or "What did you learn from your mistakes this week?" Don't be afraid to talk about failure, as it shows you're "in it" with your child and committed to problem solving collaboratively with them when things don't go well.

• *Change the way you talk to your child.* Make sure you're not speaking using "false mindset" codes, such as "You're so smart" or "You've got amazing talent," and instead use sentences like "The more you practice that piece on the piano, the more beautiful it sounds," or "When you attend all the baseball practices, you seem to enjoy the games more." Sometimes the examples come from our kids themselves. Once, when my son was in fifth or sixth grade, he said, "I had an epiphany! When you study for the test, you know the answers to the questions and it's not that hard!" I didn't know whether I was more shocked that he used the word *epiphany* in a sentence or that he made this connection himself. Throughout high school, when things got tough for him, I reminded him of his own words: When you use your brain, or practice, or do whatever it takes to increase your chances of success, you will actually increase your chances of experiencing success. And you might enjoy the *Eureka!* feeling you get when you realize you've had an epiphany.

> *The words you use can go a long way toward helping your child develop a realistic, flexible mindset.*

• *Don't jump on your child for every little thing.* Living with a child who couldn't care less can make a parent feel on edge all of the time. And what do we do when we're on edge? We overreact. All kids misbehave, but parents of kids who don't care tend to see everything as misbehavior. When a 17-year-old honor student is 10 minutes late for curfew, parents might assume it was because traffic was bad, but with a child who couldn't care less, they might assume they were late because they were smoking marijuana in the car and needed to air it out before bringing it home. Don't jump to conclusions without evidence (with the knowledge that honor students also do similar things, but they are often better at not getting caught).

• *Take care of yourself.* Check your own feelings about what's going on. Are you afraid you'll have a child who never attends college? (Reread Chapter 8 on college readiness and noncollege options to remind yourself why that's not the end of the world.) Are your expectations rooted in your own anxiety? Are you worried about what will happen to your child if she squanders all of her opportunities? Having a child who couldn't care less can be frightening, but anxiety is contagious. It can lead to kids who are paralyzed not only by their own insecurities but also by their parents' anxieties. Self-reflection can help you figure out the answers to some of these questions. Taking care of your own anxiety can set a good example for your child.

• *Sometimes there's nothing you can do in the moment, and you have to wait it out—be consciously okay with waiting.* This is a mindset that's pretty hard for most parents. We want to help our children—*now!*—but sometimes what we need to do is practice patience. Remember you're in a long-term process of growth. Growth doesn't happen in an instant. Knowing that this is part of the process can keep your anxiety in check and ultimately help foster growth.

Where to Go from Here

I wish these last two chapters were filled with lists of instructions or short-term programs that would help your child quickly become engaged, motivated, and excited to learn. Rather than relying on or looking for an instruction manual, think of this more as an evolving puzzle. The pieces to the puzzle can be found by looking at your child's APP—their aptitudes, the activities that give them pleasure, and the things they practice doing. Another piece of the puzzle relates to your expectations and whether the expectations match the goals. The questions you will want to consider include:

- Can my child do what I am asking her to do? When kids believe they can succeed, they are energized and empowered. Kids who don't care are often kids who don't believe they can be successful, because they lack the confidence, the ability, or the desire to do what they are asked to do. Things to keep in mind include:
  - When children believe their effort will lead to learning, they are more likely to expect they can succeed. If they don't believe they're capable of what you're asking them to do, no amount of coaxing will change the outcome. Success breeds success.
  - When children are appropriately supported—through encouragement and having the resources to complete tasks—they are more likely to believe they can do it and more likely to stay motivated.
  - When children know what is expected of them, and when there are clearly defined goals, they are more likely to be motivated.
  - When students receive feedback that effort makes a difference—and are shown how it makes a difference (and that it's skill focused and not ability focused), they are more likely to care.

- Parents' and teachers' expectations and attitudes shape children's expectations and attitudes about themselves. Expectations that are too high (and put too much pressure on a child) or too low ("he'll never amount to anything") influence how children think about themselves.

• Are they motivated to do what I want them to do? Do they want to do it? Here are things to keep in mind:

  - Kids tend to care more when they are engaged in activities that challenge them to grow in areas where they've already experienced some measure of success.
  - Kids who believe activities are meaningful and purposeful are more likely to become motivated.
  - Kids who find activities and academics enjoyable and interesting are more likely to care. The opposite is also true—few people care when they're asked, day after day, to do something that is not enjoyable.
  - Too many external rewards and incentives for doing something pleasurable can lead to poorer, not better, performance and motivation.
  - Relationships matter—when children interact with teachers who are enthusiastic about learning and parents who nurture their children's passions, kids are more likely to care.

• What are the barriers that are preventing my child from staying motivated? What can be done to remove these barriers? Here are the things we know can cause kids not to care. Most of these can be easily changed:

  - Too many demands on a child's time
  - Feeling that an activity isn't worth their time or not understanding why an activity is worth doing
  - Feeling unsafe or uncomfortable at school or at home
  - Schoolwork that feels unreasonable (for example, too much homework)

- Schoolwork that feels unnecessary (for example, busy work)
- Difficulty with executive function skills or other learning or emotional difficulties that make school or certain aspects of life more challenging

As the last point notes, there are some issues—depression, anxiety, learning disabilities, ADHD—that can cause some kids to just give up. The next couple of chapters provide answers to the questions of when to worry, as well as other specific issues that can get in the way of your kid caring more.

THINK, TALK, DO

 What to Think About

- How has your mindset changed over time?
- What is your child's mindset like? How has it changed over time?
- What activities do you praise in your child? How do you praise them?
- How do your child's teachers view your child? With a fixed or growth mindset? How do they praise your child?
- How does your child currently get feedback on progress?
- How have you reacted to your child's failures? Did you rush in to fix things? Get angry? Reassure your child? Do you act now like there is nothing that can be done?
- Are your expectations rooted in your own anxiety?
- Can your child do what you are asking him to do?
- Is your child motivated to do what you want her to do?
- What are the barriers that are preventing your child from caring more? What can be done to remove these barriers?

What to Talk About

Name a specific problem and ask your child:

- "What do you think would be most helpful?"
- "What didn't go well for you this week?"
- "What did you learn from your mistakes this week?"

What to Do

- Discuss with your child the power of the brain; there are resources in Chapter 12 to get you started.
- Do fun brain activities and games as a family and connect them with learning new skills.
- Change the way you praise your child, connecting praise to tangible effort and change over time.
- Be aware of your own mindset and the ways you send messages with your words and actions. Change the ones that you can.

PART IV

When You Need
Extra Help

ELEVEN

When to Worry and What to Do

Every good parent is (at least some of the time) a worried parent. I'm guessing, since you decided to read this book, that you are finding yourself more worried than usual. After reading this book, you might have come to the realization that things aren't as bad as you'd imagined. Or you might have found yourself becoming a bit more concerned. The worry might be something you can't quite put your finger on. "Yes, my child is unmotivated and couldn't care less about anything, but it's more than that," you might be thinking. This is not a book about the "more than that," but I do want to give you some direction in figuring out when "more" deserves a closer look and where to go to find answers to your questions.

Mental health concerns and learning disorders are fairly common—best estimates are that one in five children will meet criteria for a diagnosable psychological disorder at some point in their lives. Some of these "disorders" might be short lived. For example, a child might meet criteria for an anxiety disorder after a traumatic event, but then find that the symptoms end relatively quickly after treatment. Other disorders, like autism spectrum or dyslexia, can impact individuals into adulthood. Still other children have mild issues, like adjusting to a parental divorce or moving to a new school, that makes their behavior inappropriate for their age. Determining whether it's appropriate to worry or to seek additional help depends in large part on the degree to which the problem is interfering with a child's functioning.

In fact, "interfering with functioning" is the first thing you should consider when deciding how serious a problem is. One of the questions you can ask yourself is "Do my child's behaviors or symptoms interfere with his ability to do schoolwork, have friendships, or be successful in life?" If yes, you then should consider how *frequently* the behaviors happen, how *intense* the behaviors are, and how *severe* they are when they occur. Let's come back to these important concepts in a minute. First, it's important to understand what *normal* is.

The first question to ask yourself when considering the seriousness of a problem is how much the problem is interfering with your child's functioning.

Is There Such a Thing as Normal?

The short answer to this question is "It depends on how you look at it." One way to look at it is from a "How different is this child?" perspective. In other words, a child who displays too much or too little of an age-expected behavior (such as being too clingy or too aggressive) might have behaviors that would be considered outside the range of normal. For example, when I am asked to evaluate a child for symptoms of ADHD, I want to evaluate whether the child is more inattentive, impulsive, or hyperactive than a typical child his age.

Another way to look at "normal" is through a cultural lens. In this case, children who don't conform to age and culture-relevant expectations could be considered to have behaviors outside the range of normal. Some peer groups expect boys to act aggressively, so there might be a wide range of normal behavior in this area. Other cultures expect adolescents to get certain grades so they have the opportunity to attend certain types of colleges. This might lead some to conclude that being a B student means the child must have some problem with attention or a learning disability when one might not exist in a different geographical area or culture. In one case the range of normal is wider; in the other it is narrower. Either way, there will always be certain patterns of emotions, behavior, and abilities that can help determine whether there is evidence of something significant within the child that is causing distress.

From a mental health perspective, *normal* is all about "psychological well-being." Children whose behaviors are in the normal range enjoy a positive quality of life. They function well at school, at home, and with friends. Looking at this the other way, kids who have a poor quality of life, who function poorly, who don't have satisfying friendships, or who exhibit certain kinds of symptoms (see the sidebar on page 218 for more information on some of these) might have behaviors outside the normal range.

How Often? How Severe? How Much Does It Interfere?

I mentioned earlier that it's the intensity, the frequency, and the severity of the behaviors that determine whether a problem warrants further attention. Does the problem occur more than just once in a while? Are the symptoms or behaviors super intense when they occur? Do they interfere with your child's functioning? I've provided some guidelines to help you figure out the answers to these questions, but it's important for me to tell you that I've never yet had a parent say to me after the evaluation process has been completed, "I wish we'd waited longer before seeking an assessment." Many have come in saying "Why didn't I do this earlier? We would have better understood what was going on and what we could have been doing all long to help." Sometimes, when a parent comes for a consultation and there really *isn't* anything of note going on, the response can be "I can sleep better at night knowing that my kid's normal."

Here are some guidelines to help you decide whether getting support would be useful:

• *Is the behavior extreme?* I'm not talking behavior that is a bit "off." I'm talking about behaviors that you never see from other kids. If you don't notice these behaviors, perhaps other people do. Is the teacher complaining

Behaviors That Are Frequent Causes for Concern

Among the most common behaviors that are cause for concern in kids who couldn't care less are the following. Keep in mind these behaviors are only "abnormal" when they interfere with functioning, are chronic, and continue for longer than a few weeks or months.

- Difficulty paying attention at home or at school

- Poor impulse control or aggression; temper tantrums that are inappropriate for age in intensity or frequency

- Failure to respond to discipline, especially if you're being consistent about discipline

- Generally uncooperative to the point where you feel the family is constantly "walking on eggshells"

- Problems learning academic skills at school (difficulty learning to read, spell, write, or complete schoolwork) and problems completing homework

- Truancy from school, expulsions, frequent detentions

- Constant feelings of low self-esteem or feeling inferior to peers

- Problems getting along with peers or having no friends

- Feelings of sadness, depression, or anxiety

- Unusual behaviors such as talking about or experiencing implausible things, repetitive behaviors, mania, obsessive thoughts, or compulsive behaviors

about your child being behind? Disorganized? Inattentive? Impulsive? Anxious? If a lot of other people are saying "You should get these behaviors checked out," you probably should.

• *Has the problem been going on for a long time?* Is the problem chronic—does it occur almost every day (constantly anxious or daily problems with home completion) or keep reappearing (depression that is intense for a bit, then goes away and keeps coming back again)?

• *Are there a lot of symptoms* that might not seem too alarming by themselves but when put together are worrisome? For example, is your child showing signs of not caring, being anxious, *and* having difficulty learning math at school?

• *Is your child failing to progress* at the same rate as her peers? This can range from difficulty learning social skills to ability to pay attention to academic skills.

• *Are the consequences of the behaviors significant?* Has your child been using alcohol or substances? Has he been suspended from school? Does she talk about suicide or trauma? Even if these behaviors aren't chronic (in other words, you didn't know about the drug use or suicidal thoughts before), they warrant attention due to their significance.

If you answered yes to a lot of these questions, and particularly if you answered yes to the last one, seeking additional information and support is likely a good idea.

Okay, So I'm Worried . . . Now What Do I Do?

Two of the best people to consult when you're worried about your child's behavior are your child's teacher and your child's pediatrician. The pediatrician has hopefully known your child for a long time and can help you view his problems in the context of normal development and your child's own developmental trajectory. The teacher spends more time with your child than anyone except you and should be able to give you additional insight into your child's learning, social, and behavioral development. The teacher should also be able to give a perspective on whether your child's behavior is similar to that of her peers. I recommend getting as much information as possible from people you trust. If you don't have confidence in your child's current teacher or you have a new pediatrician, those might not be the best places to start. If so, start with last year's teacher, a day care provider, or a coach who knows your child well.

Your child's teacher and pediatrician are likely your best sources of additional information.

GET MORE INFORMATION

What happens after you get the feedback that more information is necessary? There are a few routes to take, and here are the options (see the next section for an explanation of the different kinds of professionals who are involved in these options):

- *Get an evaluation through the school system.* Your child is entitled to a free evaluation through your school system, regardless of your income and regardless of whether your child attends public school. The first step in this process is requesting testing (preferable in writing, but it can start with a phone call) from your school district's special education department. Once your school gets the request, it must respond within a certain period of time, which varies from state to state. There are a lot of positives to going this path. You pay nothing for the evaluation, and the services recommended by the evaluation team are provided by the school system at no cost to you. This is a good route to go if your child's issues are within the academic realm or if your child's behaviors are primarily impacting her at school. If the issues are more in the emotional realm, or if getting a clear diagnosis is important, you are better off getting a private evaluation, as school evaluations don't make diagnoses, nor do they typically thoroughly assess psychological issues such as depression or anxiety.

- *Seek an evaluation from a professional, such as a pediatric neuropsychologist, who specializes in **assessing** children for learning, attention, and developmental difficulties.* The upside to this route is that the evaluator will make a diagnosis and recommendations without regard to whether the school can provide it. You can choose the evaluator, and often the evaluation is more comprehensive. The downside is that it might take a long time to get an appointment and it may or may not be covered by insurance. (Testing is expensive, and depending on where you live, a full neuropsychological evaluation can range from a few thousand to eight thousand dollars or more. The tests used in these evaluations are expensive, and the process itself is quite time consuming for the clinician, typically taking at least 12 to 20 hours.)

• *Make an appointment with a psychologist, a psychiatrist, or another mental health professional who specializes in **treating** childhood disorders.* Your pediatrician (and sometimes your child's school) might recommend your child directly seek treatment. This route is most common when the issues are in the psychological or behavioral realm and a learning disability is not suspected. There are many types of professionals who are well qualified to administer treatments. Most frequently, these professionals are child psychologists or psychiatrists, but the title they hold is less important than the person and the experience the professional has (see below for the types of professionals you might want to consult). At a minimum, you want to make sure the professional is licensed in your state and has experience assessing or treating unmotivated kids.

SO MANY DIFFERENT PROFESSIONALS, SO FEW APPOINTMENTS

By far the biggest difficulty you will encounter after you've decided to seek an evaluation or treatment is *finding any professional* in a reasonable time frame, let alone *finding the right professional*. There is an acute shortage of mental health professionals, particularly those who specialize in children. Here's my advice: Get referrals from everyone you trust—teachers, pediatricians, other parents. Get on waiting lists. Don't be discouraged. Be persistent in letting the professionals (or more importantly, their administrative staff) know you are willing to come in for a last-minute cancellation. What professionals could be helpful? Here's a quick list:

• *Clinical psychologists* are licensed professionals who have a PhD (a doctorate of philosophy in psychology) or a PsyD (a doctorate of psychology). Both have similar training as it relates to treating and evaluating individuals, though only some have a specialization in treating children, adolescents, and families. Psychologists spend at least four years in graduate school (after completing a college degree) training in the assessment and treatment of psychological disorders. Graduate school is followed by a full-time, yearlong internship and another year of supervised postdoctoral training before they can apply for licensure.

• *Child psychologists* are psychologists who have specialized training in treating and/or assessing children. Within this field, many child psychologists specialize even further in fields such as neuropsychology, cognitive-behavioral therapy, or family therapy. You will want to make sure that the psychologist has expertise in the area that you and your child need.

• *Neuropsychologists,* mentioned above, are clinical psychologists who specialize in using neuropsychological tests to evaluate intellectual, memory, language, academic, and visual–motor skills to diagnose learning disabilities, attention problems, and developmental disorders.

• *School psychologists* are psychologists who, not surprisingly, typically work in the school setting, where they consult to classroom teachers, counsel students, and administer tests.

• *Child psychiatrists* are physicians who specialize in the diagnosis and treatment of psychological and psychiatric disorders. Psychiatrists, because they are medical doctors, can prescribe medication, whereas psychologists cannot do so in most states.

• *Other professionals* who can be helpful in getting information about your child's development are *licensed mental health counselors, speech and language therapists* (who evaluate and treat speech and language issues), *occupational therapists* (who evaluate and treat fine motor and sensory integration difficulties), and *physical therapists* (who evaluate and treat gross motor and physical functioning).

WHAT CAN YOU EXPECT FROM THE EVALUATION?

Regardless of which professional you see or whether the goal is treatment or a comprehensive assessment, the clinician will first spend time talking with you and your child. The clinician will be listening and thinking about your child's emotional, behavioral, cognitive, and social functioning as well as any situational circumstances that might be causing your child to act in a certain way. The assessment often begins with a clinical interview, which involves talking to you about why you sought treatment (in other words, your view of the problem) as well as a more detailed developmental history. Testing done within the school setting can sometimes begin by observing the child in the classroom or on the playground. Psychological testing sometimes starts with having parents and teachers fill out forms that quantify a child's behaviors.

During the clinical interview, the clinician will typically want to spend some time separately with you and with your child, as well as some time with you and your child together. The use of the term *interview* may make it sound like you're applying for a job. The use of this term is baffling to a lot of people, and it doesn't sound very warm and friendly. It's simply an appointment where you'll be asked questions about your child's development, medical history, family history, social relationships, academic history, and the expectations, fears, hopes, and concerns you have for your child. You *can*, however, think of it as a bit of an interview in the sense that you should be evaluating whether the professional is the right person for the job.

> Interview *is the right term for your initial meeting with the clinician in the sense that it's an opportunity for you to evaluate whether the clinician is the right person to assess your child.*

A good interview will focus not only on weaknesses, but also on a child's strengths and positive qualities. Interviews are most often unstructured, meaning that questions will be asked and explored in a flexible manner. While listening to what the parent is saying, the clinician will be deciding whether certain areas of functioning deserve greater exploration. The conclusion of the evaluation process should yield a better understanding of a child's particular issues in a way that directs you to the appropriate diagnosis and treatment.

WHAT KINDS OF TREATMENT ARE AVAILABLE?

Much of the answer to this question lies in what's available in your area. Some geographical areas have more resources than others. The actual treatment intervention is less important than the right person. Many studies have shown that the real magic of therapy happens within the context of a relationship between client and professional. Don't get *too* caught up in finding exactly the right kind of treatment approach (unless that is what has been specifically recommended, such as cognitive-behavioral treatment for a phobia of needles). Most experienced clinicians use a variety of techniques when working with children. That being said, the following are the kinds of treatments that are available:

• *Traditional psychotherapy*—this is sometimes called "talk therapy." If this conjures up pictures of someone lying on a couch talking about their dreams over the course of a decade, I'm happy to tell you that those sorts of treatment models are pretty rare these days. While helpful for some, most people don't have the time or money to devote to that kind of treatment. Instead, talk therapists are typically goal oriented, as well as being insight oriented. The goal is for clients to gain insight into their difficulties and for this insight to lead to changes in the problematic behaviors. This kind of therapy has been shown to be effective in treating depression, coping with life's changes (both big and small), and building better peer relationships.

• *Cognitive-behavioral therapy* (CBT) is an even more solution-focused approach. The premise of this therapy is that the way we feel about our environment and ourselves determines how we will react to it. The goals of CBT are to identify the problem behaviors or problem thoughts and replace them with more adaptive ones, to teach better coping strategies, and to help children be aware of and regulate their own behavior. CBT has been found to be effective in treating depression, anxiety, ADHD, oppositional behaviors, phobias, obsessive–compulsive disorder, posttraumatic stress disorder, and some symptoms of autism. As should be evident from this long list, CBT has been studied a lot in the last 20 years, and it's an effective treatment for many different behaviors.

• *Family therapy* is based on the idea that a child lives and grows in relationship to others, particularly family members. Unlike the therapies mentioned above, which focus on what's happening to the child as an individual, family therapists work with the entire family system. The approach assumes that some of the child's "problems" don't just reside in the child but also are determined by variables within the family. Goals of family therapy might include teaching better communication skills, helping the family identify areas of conflicts and situations that may make certain family members anxious or angry, or helping family members feel more connected to each other, while using the existing strengths of the family to help all family members handle their problems.

• *School-based services* are often the key ingredient for a child who has a learning issue or a psychological or behavioral issue that interferes with the ability to be successful in the classroom. To access school services, you need to request an evaluation and be found eligible for support. Support services can include tutoring in academic subjects, social-skills groups, behavioral support, counseling, classroom accommodations, and specialized learning environments.

• *Other treatment options* can include *medication, occupational therapy, physical therapy,* and *speech/language therapy.* Typically these kinds of options are chosen after your child has already been evaluated for one of the treatments mentioned above.

Take-Home Points

This chapter has barely skimmed the surface as to the hundreds of things parents can worry about and what can help when they do. My advice is if you're concerned, it's never a bad idea to get support from someone you trust. In addition, here are the important take-away messages:

• If you're worried, get support. Your child's pediatrician and school personnel are good places to start, and there are other professionals, such as clinical psychologists and psychiatrists, who can further evaluate any concerns as necessary.

• Finding the right clinician may take some time, and getting recommendations from people you trust, going to a reputable source such as a medical school or university psychology department, and checking the clinicians' credentials can help point you in the right direction. Training sites for psychologists and mental health counselors often provide assessment and treatment on a sliding scale. Above all, *trust your instincts*. If you don't "click" with someone, it's okay. Keep looking until you find someone who feels right.

• There's no one "perfect" treatment, and many child clinicians use more than one treatment. Regardless of the treatment, it's important to feel confident in the competence of the psychologist.

• Regardless of the treatment, it should be tailored to a child's and family's individual needs and the developmental level of the child. The treatment approach that works for a four-year-old doesn't apply to a 14-year-old.

• Regardless of the problem, whether it's a learning disability that is causing your child not to care, or depression, or anxiety, or a host of other situations, know that very good treatments are available. For some children a combination of treatments—therapy and medication, or medication and school services—work best. The most important thing to remember is to *seek treatment*.

• Your local school system can provide a wealth of support (even if your child attends a private school), but sometimes you may need to be the catalyst that makes the services "happen." You are your child's best advocate, and if you feel your child isn't getting what she needs at school, isn't making appropriate progress, or is coming home hating school, something is wrong. You should ask for an evaluation. If your child has already been evaluated, you should find out if the services that are supposed to be in place are actually being implemented.

The next chapter offers sources of much more information about each one of the topics covered in this chapter and the rest of the book.

TWELVE

Resources

General Parenting

BOOKS

Clear, J. (2018). *Atomic Habits: An Easy and Proven Way to Build Good Habits & Break Bad Ones*. London, UK: Penguin.

Eidens, A. (2018). *Big Life Journal: Teen Edition*. Stamford, CT: Eidens.

Hibbs, B. J., & Rostain, A. (2019). *The Stressed Years of Their Lives: Helping Your Child Survive and Thrive During Their College Years*. New York: St. Martin's Press.

Lahey, J. (2015). *The Gift of Failure: How the Best Parents Learn to Let Go So Their Children Can Succeed*. New York: Harper Collins.

Levine, M. (2021). *Ready or Not: Preparing Our Kids to Thrive in an Uncertain and Rapidly Changing World*. New York: HarperCollins.

Lythcott-Haims, J. (2015). *How to Raise an Adult: Break Free of the Overparenting Trap and Prepare Your Kid for Success*. New York: Henry Holt.

McCready, A. (2016). *The Me, Me, Me Epidemic: A Step-by-Step Guide to Raising Capable, Grateful Kids in an Over-Entitled World*. New York: TarcherPerigee.

Siegel, D. J., & Bryson, T. P. (2012). *The Whole-Brain Child: 12 Revolutionary Strategies to Nurture Your Child's Developing Mind* (illustrated ed.). New York: Bantam.

Stixrud, W., & Johnson, N. (2019). *The Self-Driven Child: The Science and Sense of Giving Your Kids More Control Over Their Lives*. London, UK: Penguin.

Stixrud, W., & Johnson, N. (2021). *What Do You Say?: How to Talk with Kids to Build Motivation, Stress Tolerance, and a Happy Home*. New York: Viking.

Weissbourd, R. (2010). *The Parents We Mean to Be: How Well-Intentioned Adults Undermine Children's Moral and Emotional Development*. Boston: Houghton Mifflin Harcourt.

WEBSITES

Positive Parenting: *www.cdc.gov/ncbddd/childdevelopment/positiveparenting*
Positive Psychology: *https://positivepsychology.com/goal-setting-exercises*
Wish, Outcome, Obstacle, Pain: *https://woopmylife.org*

More Help for When You Are Worried

GENERAL BOOKS ON MENTAL HEALTH

Braaten, E. (2011). *How to Find Mental Health Care for Your Child*. Washington, DC: American Psychological Association.
Braaten, E., & Felopulos, G. (2004). *Straight Talk about Psychological Testing for Kids*. New York: Guilford Press.
Wilens, T. E. (2016). *Straight Talk about Psychiatric Medications for Kids* (4th ed.). New York: Guilford Press.

CHILD MENTAL HEALTH WEBSITES

Effective Child Therapy: *https://effectivechildtherapy.org*
The Clay Center for Young Healthy Minds: *www.mghclaycenter.org*

ADHD

Books

Barkley, R. (2020). *Taking Charge of ADHD: The Complete, Authoritative Guide for Parents* (4th ed.). New York: Guilford Press.
Hallowell, E. M., & Ratey, J. J. (2011). *Driven to Distraction: Recognizing and Coping with Attention Deficit Disorder from Childhood through Adulthood*. New York: Anchor Books.
Nigg, J. T. (2017). *Getting Ahead of ADHD: What Next-Generation Science Says about Treatments That Work—and How You Can Make Them Work for Your Child*. New York: Guilford Press.

Websites

ADDitude: Inside the ADHD Mind: *www.additudemag.com*
Children and Adults with Attention-Deficit/Hyperactivity Disorder: *https://chadd.org*

ANXIETY

Books

Chansky, T. (2014). *Freeing Your Child from Anxiety: Practical Strategies to Overcome Fears, Worries, and Phobias and Be Prepared for Life—from Toddlers to Teens.* New York: Harmony.

Dacey, J. S., & Fiore, L. B. (2000). *Your Anxious Child: How Parents and Teachers Can Relieve Anxiety in Children.* San Francisco, CA: Jossey-Bass.

Khanna, M. S., Ledley, D. R., & Chansky, T. (2018). *The Worry Workbook for Kids: Helping Children to Overcome Anxiety and the Fear of Uncertainty.* Oakland, CA: New Harbinger Publications.

Nelson, M. K. (2012). *Parenting Out of Control: Anxious Parents in Uncertain Times.* New York University Press.

Rapee, R. M. (2008). *Helping Your Anxious Child: A Step-by-Step Guide for Parents.* Oakland, CA: New Harbinger Publications.

Wilson, R., & Lyons, L. (2013). *Anxious Kids, Anxious Parents: 7 Ways to Stop the Worry Cycle and Raise Courageous and Independent Children.* Deerfield Beach, FL: Health Communications.

Websites

Coping Cat Parents: OCD and Anxiety Institute: *www.copingcatparents.com*

WorryWiseKids Children's Center for OCD and Anxiety: *http://worrywisekids.org*

Project YES (Youth Empowerment and Support) at the Lab for Scalable Mental Health: *www.schleiderlab.org/yes.html*

DEPRESSION

Empfield, M., & Bakalar, N. (2001). *Understanding Teenage Depression: A Guide to Diagnosis, Treatment, and Management.* New York: Henry Holt.

Koplewicz, H. (2003). *More Than Moody: Recognizing and Treating Adolescent Depression.* New York: Perigee.

Seligman, M. E. P., Reivich, K., Jaycox, L., & Gillham, J. (2007). *The Optimistic Child: A Proven Program to Safeguard Children Against Depression and Build Lifelong Resilience.* Boston: Houghton Mifflin.

Wright, J. H., & McCray, L. W. (2012). *Breaking Free from Depression: Pathways to Wellness.* New York: Guilford Press.

EXECUTIVE FUNCTION

Dawson, P., & Guare, R. (2009). *Smart but Scattered: The Revolutionary "Executive Skills" Approach to Helping Kids Reach Their Potential.* New York: Guilford Press.

Delman, M. (2018). *Your Kid's Gonna Be Okay: A Guide to Raising Competent and Confident Kids.* Needham, MA: Beyond Booksmart.

Gallagher, R., Spira, E. G., & Rosenblatt, J. L. (2018). *The Organized Child: An Effective Program to Maximize Your Kid's Potential—in School and in Life.* New York: Guilford Press.

Josel, L. (2020). *How to Do It Now Because It's Not Going Away: An Expert Guide to Getting Stuff Done.* Minneapolis, MN: Zest Books.

Morgenstern, J. (2018). *Time to Parent: Organizing Your Life to Bring Out the Best in Your Child and You.* New York: Henry Holt.

Pinsky, S. C. (2012). *Organizing Solutions for People with ADHD.* Gloucester, MA: Fair Winds.

LEARNING DIFFERENCES

Books

Braaten, E., & Willoughby, B. (2014). *Bright Kids Who Can't Keep Up.* New York: Guilford Press.

Flink, D. (2014). *Thinking Differently: An Inspiring Guide for Parents of Children with Learning Disabilities.* New York: William Morrow.

Shaywitz, S. E. (2020). *Overcoming Dyslexia* (2nd ed.). New York: Alfred A. Knopf.

Websites

Council for Exceptional Children: *https://exceptionalchildren.org*
Learning Disabilities Association of America: *https://ldaamerica.org*
National Center for Learning Disabilities: *www.ncld.org*
The Neurodiversity University: *https://neurodiversitypodcast.com*
Q.E.D. Foundation: Competency-Based Learning: *https://allkindsofminds.org*
Tilt Parenting: "Differently Wired": *https://tiltparenting.com*
Understood: Learning and Thinking Differences: *www.understood.org*

Special Topics

ACADEMIC SUPPORT

Books

Bay-Williams, J., & Kling, G. (2019). *Math Fact Fluency: 60+ Games and Assessment Tools to Support Learning and Retention.* Alexandria, VA: ASCD.

Rasinski, T. V., & Smith, M. C. (2021). *The Megabook of Fluency.* New York: Scholastic Professional.

Websites

BrainPOP: Interactive/Entertaining Help: *https://jr.brainpop.com*
Khan Academy Kids Online Tutoring Resource: *https://learn.khanacademy.org/khan-academy-kids*
Learning Without Tears: *www.lwtears.com*
Reading Rockets: *www.readingrockets.org*

GOAL SETTING

Duckworth, A. (2018). *Grit: The Power of Passion and Perseverance.* New York: Scribner.
George, M. (2020). *Smart Goals, Smart Me: A Goal Setting Planner and Journal.* Sweden: Pink Elephant Publications.
Hyatt, M. (2018). *Your Best Year Ever: A 5-Step Plan For Achieving Your Most Important Goals.* Grand Rapids, MI: Baker Books.

SLEEP

Books

Canapari, C. (2019). *It's Never Too Late to Sleep Train: The Low-Stress Way to High-Quality Sleep for Babies, Kids, and Parents.* New York: Harmony/Rodale.
Kurcinka, M. S. (2009). *Sleepless in America: Is Your Child Misbehaving . . . or Missing Sleep?* New York: HarperCollins.

Website

Sleep Foundation: Children and Sleep: *www.sleepfoundation.org/children-and-sleep*

GROWTH MINDSET

Books

Dweck, C. (2016). *Mindset: The New Psychology of Success.* New York: Random House.
Hardy, B. (2018). *Willpower Doesn't Work: Discover the Hidden Keys to Success.* New York: Hachette Books.

Website

Growth Mindset Institute: *www.growthmindsetinstitute.org*

OVERSCHEDULING

Abeles, V. (2015). *Beyond Measure: Rescuing an Overscheduled, Overtested, Underestimated Generation*. New York: Simon & Schuster.

Payne, K. J., & Ross, L. M. (2020). *Simplicity Parenting: Using the Extraordinary Power of Less to Raise Calmer, Happier, and More Secure Kids*. New York: Ballantine Books.

PERSONALITY TRAITS

Books

Barron, B., & Tieger, P. D. (1997). *Nurture by Nature: Understand Your Child's Personality Type—and Become a Better Parent*. New York: Little Brown & Company.

Waters, L. (2017). *The Strength Switch: How The New Science of Strength-Based Parenting Can Help Your Child and Your Teen to Flourish*. New York: Avery.

Website

Values in Action Inventory: *www.viacharacter.org*

SOCIAL MEDIA

Books

Carr, N. G. (2010). *The Shallows: What the Internet Is Doing to Our Brains*. New York: W.W. Norton.

Gold, J. (2015). *Screen-Smart Parenting: How to Find Balance and Benefit in Your Child's Use of Social Media, Apps, and Digital Devices*. New York: Guilford Press.

Miner, J. (2019). *Raising a Screen-Smart Kid: Embrace the Good and Avoid the Bad in the Digital Age*. New York: TarcherPerigee.

Steiner-Adair, C., & Barker, T. H. (2014). *The Big Disconnect: Protecting Childhood and Family Relationships in the Digital Age*. New York: HarperCollins.

Website

Family Media Planning: *www.healthychildren.org/English/media*

Index

About the Author

Ellen Braaten, PhD, is Executive Director of the Learning and Emotional Assessment Program at Massachusetts General Hospital, Associate Professor of Psychology at Harvard Medical School, and Visiting Professor at Charles University in Prague, Czech Republic. Dr. Braaten is an internationally recognized expert on neuropsychological and psychological assessment of children, particularly in the areas of learning and attention difficulties. She has published numerous books for professionals and parents, including *Bright Kids Who Can't Keep Up*.